The Three-Pound Enigma

The Three-Pound Enigma

The Human Brain and the Quest to Unlock Its Mysteries

by Shannon Moffett

ALGONQUIN BOOKS OF CHAPEL HILL | 2006

Published by
Algonquin Books of Chapel Hill
Post Office Box 2225
Chapel Hill, North Carolina 27515-2225

a division of
Workman Publishing
708 Broadway
New York, New York 10003

Quotation by Bob Stickgold on page 129, line 4, reprinted from a book
manuscript in preparation, with permission from the author.

Poem on page 268 reprinted from Norman Fischer, *On Whether or Not to
Believe in Your Mind* (Great Barrington, MA: The Figures, 1987), with
permission from the author and the publisher.

Library of Congress Cataloging-in-Publication Data
Moffett, Shannon, 1972–
    The three-pound enigma : the human brain and the quest to unlock
its mysteries / by Shannon Moffett.
        p. cm.
    Includes bibliographical references and index.
    ISBN-13: 978-1-56512-423-3
    ISBN-10: 1-56512-423-5
    1. Brain—Popular works.   2. Brain—Localization of functions—
Popular works.   I. Title.
QP376.M5845 2005
612.8'2—dc22   2005048283

10 9 8 7 6 5 4 3 2 1
First Edition

This book is dedicated to four doctors and one nurse
who kept me healthy enough to write it.

SH

FM

MW

CC

AJ

Contents

Acknowledgments   *ix*

Introduction   *1*

    PRELUDE: Postconception   *4*

1   Touching the Brain   *7*

    INTERLUDE: Embryonic Period   *39*

2   Watching the Brain   *43*

    INTERLUDE: Fetal Period   *63*

3   Mining the Brain   *66*

    INTERLUDE: Childhood   *109*

4   The Dreaming Brain   *111*

    INTERLUDE: Adolescence   *144*

5   Multiple Minds   *147*

    INTERLUDE: Adulthood   *184*

6   Mind and Magic   *190*

    INTERLUDE: Old Age   *222*

7   Open Mind   *227*

    INTERLUDE: Death   *253*

8   Mind and Body   *257*

Sources   *279*

Illustration Credits   *297*

Index   *299*

| Acknowledgments

BEN BARRES DESIGNED the course that inspired this book and answered the random questions I sent his way as I was writing it: I thank him for both. Undying gratitude to Stanford University School of Medicine and to Audrey Shafer and the Arts and Humanities Medical Scholars Committee for the money and support to start this project. Thanks to Rona Giffard for advising me through the first stages, to Ann Banchoff and Malcolm Gladwell for early encouragement, and to Elissa May Meites for reading early drafts. Thanks to Allan Hobson for agreeing to be a subject early on. When I sent the first two chapters to Laurence Gonzales, he actually read them and passed them on, which got the whole thing started. Thanks to Marianne Merola, my agent, and Antonia Fusco, my editor, who slogged through it all with me. Enormous thanks to Paul and Florence Libin, Astro and Zoe and Willow Teller, and especially Dave Andre for the above-and-beyond-the-call-of-duty hospitality. Roger Nicoll gave me Robert Malinow, who agreed to be a subject and just as gracefully agreed not to be a subject, and Idee Mallardi set up housing for that ill-fated trip to Cold Springs Harbor, for which I thank them all. Elliott Wolfe set up endless directed readings without any complaint, and Marti Trujillo dealt with my bizarre financial aid situation as I completed this book. Thanks to Gary Glover for explaining fMRI and then re-explaining it after reading my first attempt. Thanks to Naomi Quesada and Justin Ramos for transcription, to Ray Balise for reading and commenting on the entire manuscript, and to Raymond Sobel for promptly and thoroughly answering a stranger's eleventh-hour question about neurodevelopment. Eternal thanks to each of the subjects for agreeing to the extended and invasive interview process, and for reading and correcting drafts as they were written. Any errors that remain are my own.

This book would have been impossible without the support and patience of my friends and family—Natalie and all the Pagelers (who seemed to have no problem with my dropping off the face of the earth for months at a time, then showing up on their doorstep with no no-tice), Molly Purves and Sarah K. Lippmann (who've shown a similar forbearance), Andrea Libin, queen of the extended phone call and high priestess of our cult of the exhaustively explored nuance, John High and Sascha, my mom (Nancy Moffett, who, when I was eight, taught me to say "Gertrude, whose teeth were falling out and who an-swered the door leaning on her cane" instead of "the old woman") and my dad (Tom Moffett, who taught me that "enormous" is spelled "b-i-g"), Solveig Nielsen (whom I'd travel a long way to see even if she didn't give me cigarettes and her osso bucco weren't so good), and my younger sister, Maggie, whom I miss every day and is the one per-son I'll go to when no one understands. And then there's Michael Choy, who read it all even when he didn't have to, who held my hand and my head, tucked me in and cooked for me and washed the dishes and waited up late and woke up early and accepted the fact that I haven't had a true day off since we sat in that garish Paris Internet café and found out—a week after the fact—that the book had sold. Af-ter all the research and philosophizing I still don't know what a self or a soul is, but I know I love him with all of mine.

| Introduction

I FIRST SAW A HUMAN brain in gross anatomy, during the early weeks of medical school. My dissecting partner and I had cut apart most of our cadaver by then: we'd pulled out her lungs, dislocated her shoulder to see the slick yellow ball of the humerus inside it, held her heart in our hands. But still, her face—the eyes someone once looked into with love, the mouth she had used to smile and sob, the eyebrows she would have raised in surprise—was intact. Our job that day was to use a handsaw to cut through her skull above those eyebrows. It was strenuous, slippery, and gruesome work, and we were grimly serious by the time we had finished and could turn back the top of her head, like a cap, to reveal her brain, sitting behind the bridge of her nose on a sort of shelf made by the convergence of the five main bones of her skull. The brain was a murky brown, and when we touched it, it was firm, like a block of cheese. We snipped it from her spinal cord and removed it from her skull.

As far as science can tell, that lump of tissue had held the series of connections and feelings, associations and impressions, that had been this woman. But where was her mind now? When we had first unwrapped the formalin-soaked cloth covering her hands, we'd found our cadaver's fingernails still wore a perfect coat of light purple polish. Did this woman's taste for lavender survive the death of her body? Was it contained in the brain I now held, frozen there? It didn't seem possible. Yet neither did her mind's complete extinction. Did her loves and disappointments and memories exist somewhere still, or had they died when her body did?

It may have been at that moment in the anatomy lab that I first became fascinated with the brain and its relationship to the mind. Or maybe it wasn't until our neurobiology class a few weeks later. Over nine weeks we heard some sixteen scholars speak on different topics, usually one in which they themselves were doing research, in which case we were treated to a passionate discourse on that aspect of the mind or brain.

Dr. John Gabrieli, featured in this book, described what he and others have learned about memory and amnesia. Dr. William Newsome, who studies macaque monkeys, told us what he had learned about vision—the best understood of all our five senses—from the study of primates' brains. And Dr. Allan Basbaum presented his research into pain. He taught us that pain is subjective—that fear, mental associations like memories, and the context in which a painful stimulus is felt can all heighten (or reduce) the experience of pain in ways that remain mysterious. No one knows, he told us, why women who give birth alone and without prenatal care experience much more pain during labor than well-prepared women with good family support. In colored chalk, he then rendered a drawing in the style of Piet Mondrian, like this:

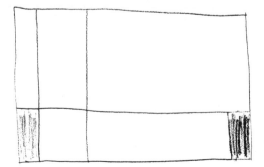

Why is it, he asked, that some of us look at a Mondrian and shrug our shoulders, wondering what's for lunch, while others who know art and are familiar with Mondrian's artistic development might break into tears, stunned at the beautiful simplicity he achieved after years of reduction?

All of this led to Basbaum's unforgettable statement: "No one knows where exactly in the brain the perception of pain is located," he said, "but I'll tell you this: when they find out where beauty is located, pain will be right next door."

These were big ideas, with new concepts presented by the people living these questions daily. It occurred to me that there was no reason this kind of learning should be limited to medical students. The big questions in neuroscience—Where is memory? How do we see? What happens when we think?—are still being sorted out, and much of what we were being taught seemed relevant to daily life, to things we had all wondered about in idle moments. So I began writing a series of profiles, each containing two portraits—one of a person, the other of the brain or mind from that person's perspective. All of those profiled here are devoted to grappling with one particular mystery related to the mind, recognizing that any solution will only present new questions.

I have done my best to provide context for each person's work and to provide connections between the chapters but have also tried to leave space for different interpretations, for the one hundred billion neurons in your brain to create new connections, reach new conclusions. Those connections and conclusions will be different from my own, a fact that reflects many of the mysteries described here.

Conception	6 weeks	10 weeks	30 weeks	6 years	Adolescence	Adulthood	Old Age	Death

Birth

When you were a three-week-old embryo, your neural tube—the part of you that would become your brain and your spinal cord—would have looked, if anyone had checked you out under an electron microscope, like a cannoli shell:

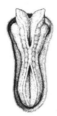

As you developed over the next day or two, that cannoli became more tubelike, as if someone were pinching the pastry closed, starting at the center and moving out toward the ends:

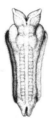

By the time you were twenty-four days old, your neural tube (pictured below from the side) had a lumpy bulge at the top:

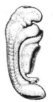

Over the next week, two parts of that topmost bulge began grow-ing rapidly, at the same time curving until they looked like two beans (they were like beans in shape, at least—at the time, your entire body was about half the size of a lima bean):

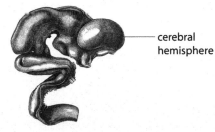

cerebral hemisphere

Those two mini beans appeared a little more than a month after you were conceived, so it's possible that at the time, no one knew you ex-isted. But over the next couple of months, those bean-shaped swellings kept growing. As they grew, their surfaces started to buckle and wrinkle. They continued enlarging and wrinkling until just before you were born, at which point they had enveloped most of the top of your neural tube. Those beans became, of course, your cerebral hemispheres.

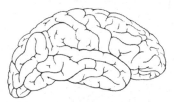

In a fully developed human brain, each cerebral hemisphere is di-vided into five lobes, four of which can be seen from the outside: the frontal lobe, the parietal lobe, the occipital lobe, and the temporal lobe:*

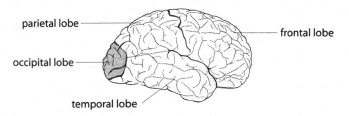

parietal lobe

frontal lobe

occipital lobe

temporal lobe

*The fifth lobe, the limbic lobe, is on the inside surface of each cerebral hemi-sphere.

Those lobes make up the cerebral cortex, and their outer surface is the gray matter—a misnomer, since gray matter in a living brain is really a lucent pink. In humans, almost all the gray matter of the hemispheres is neocortex, believed to have evolved more recently than two other bits of cerebral cortex: the paleocortex, a half-dollar-size area on the underside of the hemispheres, and the archicortex, buried within the temporal lobes at the sides of the brain. In a healthy, living brain, the gray matter in all those areas has a consistency about like that of tapioca pudding.

The parts of your neural tube enveloped by your cerebral hemispheres became the thalamus (a sort of central switching station for information coming into and leaving your brain) and other deep-brain structures. The structures not entirely covered by your cerebrum turned into the cerebellum (whose name means "little brain")—which helps in coordinating movement—and the brain stem. The brain stem is crucial for many of our basic living needs; it keeps us breathing and keeps our hearts beating.

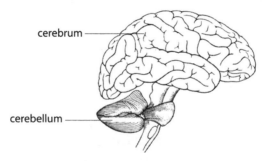

The cerebral hemispheres, deep-brain structures, cerebellum, and brain stem are all encased in the skull, that bony armor protecting the fragile, wrinkly, puddinglike blob that, as far as we know, is *you*—the seat of every hope, dream, fear, memory, capability, characteristic, idea, emotion, thought, plan, potential action, and conscious experience that makes you who you are.

Knowing nothing is a great place to start. I hope you end up there.

—NORMAN FISCHER

1 | Touching the Brain

"SEE THAT BULLET OVER THERE?" Dr. Roberta Glick asks, moving aside so I can look over her shoulder. "You don't ever want to pull something directly out of the brain—it's like pulling your finger out of a dam." It's 5:00 p.m. on a Saturday, and we are in an operating room at Chicago's Cook County Hospital. As the attending neurosurgeon on call, Glick is responsible for removing the bullet, which is lodged in the head of a man we met early this morning.

To Glick's left is Dr. Mike Song, the chief neurosurgical resident, who is impatient to get started. Less than an hour ago, as Glick was in her station wagon, barreling along Lake Shore Drive in her second trip to the hospital today, she called Song and instructed him to wait for her arrival before beginning what they consider to be the actual surgery. He complied, but when we walked into the OR moments ago, he was already well into what any layperson would consider surgery: wearing a mask, gown, and gloves wet with the patient's blood, he is standing behind the head of the operating table. High above it is a kitchen-table-size tray of instruments swathed in sterile blue drapes, attended by the scrub nurse in a blue sterile gown, cap, and mask. On the other side of the table is another drape, hung perpendicular to the floor, behind which crouch the anesthesiologists, invisible to me and silent as they keep the patient in the delicate place between sleep and death. In front of us, the patient himself is nothing but a swatch of flesh the size of a softball in a sea of blue. The skin of his scalp is open like a red mouth, exposing a glistening ellipse of white skull, near one edge of which is the flattened gray lump that is the bullet.

I'D MET GLICK before dawn at a Starbucks in Evanston, the affluent suburb just north of Chicago where she lives with her husband and two sons. She was fifteen minutes late because Daniel, her nine-year-old, had slammed his finger in a door. "I had to stay and ice it. He was crying, poor kid," she told me as we joined the line in front of the barista. There was nothing in Glick's tone or appearance to indicate to the morning coffee crowd that she ever sees an injury more traumatic or life threatening than the bruising of her son's finger.

Solidly built, with waist-length red hair, wearing beaten-metal earrings dangling almost to her shoulders and a saffron batik dress ("I buy all my clothes at art fairs"), Glick looked like someone you'd expect to find reading storybooks to kindergartners in a public library, rather than performing neurosurgery in an inner-city public hospital. But at forty-eight, she has been a practicing neurosurgeon for twenty-three years. Her specialty is brain tumors, and her research is aimed at finding new ways to combat brain cancer, but she also treats congenital malformations of the brain and its blood vessels, as well as the brain injuries so common at Cook County, a hospital known for its trauma unit, the poverty of its patients, and the dedication of the doctors who serve them.

Latte in hand, Glick got in her car for the first of her two trips to the hospital that day. She'd told me on the phone the day before that the past week had been crazy. And because she graduated from high school at sixteen years old and then went on to college and double majored (in molecular biology and psychology) and triple minored (in music, art, and chemistry) and then went to graduate school for a PhD in neuroanatomy and then to medical school and was a resident in what is widely agreed to be the most punishing of medical specialties and now raises two children while working fifty to sixty hours a week as a neurosurgeon, I believed her.

Between bites of yogurt ("I haven't eaten since, like, three o'clock yesterday"), she told me more about the last few days. During that time the mother of a friend had died, although as Glick tells it, that was the most life-affirming of recent events: "I mean, she's seen all of life." But then after the funeral, "it was just like this week of drama." On Saturday she'd gone to a bar mitzvah at which two different friends approached her to discuss finding care for their terminally ill family members. "And Sunday it was the guy with the brain tumor's son."

At the time there were actually several guys with brain tumors in Glick's life outside the hospital. Three of her longtime friends were suffering from terminal brain cancer and had sought her out to help them understand what was happening to them. And so, after a day of treating patients at work with serious brain disease, many of them with cancer, Glick often spent hours visiting or on the phone with one or another of her friends with cancer, giving medical advice but also simply support. "I've turned into a cheerleader," she said. "I'm the rah-rah for people with brain tumors."

The previous Sunday, one of these friends, a man in his mid-forties, had died, leaving behind his wife and two young children, who go to school with Glick's sons. Glick had spent that afternoon with his older boy. "When he died, his son said, 'I have to talk to Roberta — she can tell me what happened.' So I went over there and showed him all the MRIs, talked to him about how sometimes some cells in your brain can go crazy and start growing out of control. I told him it was kind of like *Alien*, with this thing inside you. It was the only analogy I could think of."

Although Glick has to do that sort of thing every day, the thought of explaining cancer to a nine-year-old, in the context of the death of his own father, silenced me. She knew what I was thinking. "People are always like, 'How do you make sense of this tragedy?'" she said. "How I make sense of it is—" At that point she stopped to use her sleeve to mop up some moisture collecting on her windshield.

A conversation with Glick is like a ride on a roller coaster: it's fast, it takes unexpected twists and turns, and steering it isn't an option. When she'd finished with the windshield, Glick was thinking about the use of quantitative measurements in determining surgical outcomes, so that's what we talked about. "The scientific method of today has become almost antihuman," she said. Particularly within neurosurgery, and particularly in regard to brain tumors, Glick thinks the focus of medicine is too much on extension of life rather than on the quality of the life that's been extended. "It's all about survival, progression-free survival," she said, rather than about more qualitative measures like the ability of patients to take care of themselves or enjoy life. Glick herself has only recently come to this realization as she's watched her friends deteriorate, unable to do things that had given them joy before their illnesses, yet kept alive with surgeries and chemotherapy.

Kept alive for a while, at least. Glick did eventually return to the topic of how she understood her friend's death. "There's this Jewish mysticism thing where you put God at the center," she said. "But I transform it so that you put your friend at the center, and you think of all the people whose lives he affects as coming off like spokes. If you try to make sense out of something so tragic—this person enabled all these other people to do good things. They made meals for the family or called them. It affected lives in so many ways."

Glick, who was not raised a religious Jew, has been doing what she calls "private spiritual study"—which encompasses everything from Torah to kabbalistic thought—for a decade, and was bat mitzvahed two years before I met her. But there was no time to talk further about that. "Oh, look at the sun," she said. It was foggy ahead of us, but on our left the early-morning sun sent out a fan of light from behind a bank of silver cloud. It hit the surface of Lake Michigan and ignited it to a dazzling pool of fire. "It's like *rays*. You have to see it through these glasses," she said, and gave me her sunglasses.

Even with the glasses, I knew I could never truly share her vision, since Glick sees nature through the lens of her lifelong fascination with the brain. During that same drive, she listed things she thinks look like brains, which include popcorn, walnuts ("now that's brain food") and trees in winter ("I love the trees without leaves. The trees without leaves look like neural networks to me, beautiful and lacy").

Of course, Glick isn't the first to compare neurons to trees. The short projections that extend from the cell body of a neuron are known as dendrites, from the Greek word for "tree," and the long, trunklike axon that comes off the other side of the cell body is often said to "arborize" into branches.

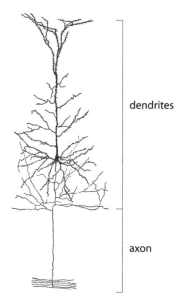

dendrites

axon

© by Ramon y Cajal's heirs

The comparison has been unavoidable since the cells were first seen clearly under the microscope. But over a hundred years after that first sighting (by an Italian named Camillo Golgi) and almost twenty years after the end of her own training, that Glick still finds the comparison fresh enough to think about during her morning commute is remarkable. "I see the brain everywhere," she told me, and indeed, when we got to her office, I spied a picture tacked to her bulletin board of a species of lichen she had found and photographed on a hike in New Mexico; it looks for all the world like a cerebral hemisphere lying amid the scrub brush.

The office in which that picture hangs is an eight-by-ten cubby, carpeted in burnt orange. Into that space Glick has crammed two desks (one of which now holds a computer, something she'd done without until well into the twenty-first century), a couch, two towering filing cabinets, and an old set of glass-front bookcases. There are Asian tapestries on the walls, a bouquet of white coats—some a little the worse for wear—hanging on the back of the door, and a poster advertising the seventeenth annual Rally Against Handgun Violence. Surgical textbooks and journal papers are everywhere—on the shelves, in rows and stacks on top of the filing cabinets, balanced on the back of the couch. Scores of clippings and photos, notes, and sketches all but obscure the whiteboard above the computer. "Think of it as a patchwork quilt," Glick said when she caught me checking out her office. "I have it all, but I have too much of it all."

We stopped just long enough for Glick to put down her purse—an ancient Coach bag, worn and bulging at the seams—the strap of which holds her beeper (when she's out of the hospital) and a hair clip. She hung the beeper from the neck of her dress, where it lives when she's in the hospital but not doing surgery, and went to check on her patients.

We started by visiting Song in the residents' on-call room, a tiny, stifling, windowless closet barely big enough for a bunk bed, a small table, and a shelf of X-rays and CT scans in huge manila folders. Song put a few CTs on a light box on the wall; they showed the head of the man I would later watch them operate on, the bullet a dark spot at the back of his skull. As they reviewed the images, Song, whose job entailed spending six days a week and every other night in the hospital, munched on some stale-looking chocolate chip cookies. The neurosurgeon Frank Vertosick has written that "a chief resident never finishes a workday, he just sort of amputates it." Song looked as if last night's amputation had been unsuccessful, but when they decided the patient needed surgery, he wanted to get it done as soon as possible. "You wanna do him today?" Glick asked. "We'll do him later—I have to go to temple."

Song, who's Korean, agreed. "I'll have to cancel my bar mitzvah, though," he said, and Glick screamed with laughter. That kind of joke has a particular resonance at Cook County, where most of the patients are of a different nationality from their doctors, and most of the doctors are of different nationalities from one another. Earlier that week, Glick and I had walked past a group of medical students, residents, and doctors congregated outside a patient's room; the group included a yarmulke, a turban, a headscarf, dreadlocks, and every skin color imaginable. "Like a meeting of the UN," Glick said.

From the on-call room, Glick went next to the neurosurgical intensive care unit, across the hall, a narrow rectangle with beds along both long sides and an aisle in the middle serving the constant traffic of doctors and nurses. There she saw, in rapid succession, a man who'd been in a brawl and immediately afterward a car accident; a man who'd fallen off a porch, broken his neck, and since spent more than a month in the hospital catching infection after infection; a man whose sky-high blood pressure had caused an artery in his brain to burst; and a man Glick had operated on for a pituitary tumor the day before.

At each patient's bed, Glick shrieked, "Hello Mr. ——, can you hear me?" If the patient didn't make some kind of noise in response, she'd take his hand and, at the top of her lungs, ask him to squeeze. It's a ritual that's hard to get used to: when you walk into a room full of the gravely ill, lying in beds and hooked up to monitors and ventilators, your first impulse is to be very, very quiet. But Glick said, "If they're able to listen and follow commands, that's like a big thing." The ability to hear and respond bodes well for a patient's recovery, indicating that the brain's sensory and cognitive function is intact. Which makes it important for Glick to ensure that a lack of response from one of her patients isn't due to a soft voice that fails to penetrate the low-level racket caused by all those machines and the nurses' conversations.

That day, the only patient who was able to do much more than squeeze Glick's hand was the man who'd had the pituitary tumor removed. He told her that his vision was better since his operation. This operation—which Glick sometimes refers to as "picking the berry," because the pituitary gland looks like one—involves accessing the brain from underneath. She does this by peeling up the skin of the patient's face behind their upper lip and then drilling through the two thin layers of bone that separate the cavity behind the nose from the brain. The pituitary gland, which is responsible for secreting a number of hormones, lies just above that spot, dangling from a stalk that communicates with the hypothalamus gland, deeper in the brain.

Just in front of that stalk, the optic nerves cross on their way from the eyes to the brain. After the crossing, known as the optic chiasm, each nerve (now technically known as a tract, to signal that beyond the chiasm it is considered a part of the brain) travels alongside the stalk and above the pituitary gland itself, then alongside the thalamus, that switching station for information to and from the brain. At the back of each thalamus, both optic tracts separate into numerous fibers that fan out and make their way to the occipital lobe, at the very back of the brain, which is where visual information from the retina begins to be processed.

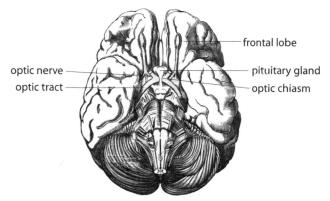

optic nerve
optic tract
frontal lobe
pituitary gland
optic chiasm

This is the brain seen from the underside, with the front of the brain toward the top of the page.

If the pituitary grows, as it does when some of its cells become cancerous, the pressure it exerts on the optic chiasm above it can effectively shut down both optic nerves by blocking the passage of information along them from the eye to the back of the brain. This pinching leads to blindness, although sometimes vision can be saved if the tumor is removed early enough, before the nerve damage is irreparable.

How much of this man's sight would return was still in question. Glick had said earlier that she thought he might need another operation, as she wasn't sure they'd been able to get much of the tumor out. For now, though, he was smiling, as was his wife, relief at having the operation over with written across their faces.

After the ICU, Glick and Song went to "the floor," regular hospital rooms for patients who don't need the close, round-the-clock monitoring in the ICU. The floor at Cook County consisted of gray hallways lined with pink partitions of the sort you might find separating the stalls in a public bathroom. Each gap in the partitions led to a patient cubicle. The cubicles contained two beds, a space between for a doctor and a couple of associates to squeeze in, and not much else. Once we were all inside the first cubicle, I could barely see the patient, a Latino man sitting on the edge of his cot, awake and alert, grinning like what he was—a guy who'd narrowly escaped death. Here was the patient whose CTs we'd looked at in the on-call room and whose scalp I would see laid open later that day.

The patient had been brought in after he was shot in the head two nights before. At that time, the residents had left the bullet in place. This course of action is fairly routine; Glick told me the best way to treat a gunshot wound (or GSW, as they're known at places like Cook County, where they're common enough to require abbreviation) to the head is often to leave the bullet in the brain. In many cases, she said, the bullet will shatter upon hitting the bone of the skull. The pieces of bullet then break off shards of skull, driving them into the brain as well. With so many bits of bone and metal lodged individually in the brain, the probing involved in going after each piece could ultimately cause more damage than the initial injury. Nevertheless, before the development of antibiotics, that probing was necessary, as each fragment, contaminated with dirt, hair, skin, and bacteria, could serve as the nidus for a brain infection. Since the development of antibiotics, however, research has shown that it is now unnecessary, and in fact detrimental, to chase down small foreign bodies in the brain following a traumatic injury. Today, surgeons usually take out larger pieces and trust to antibiotics to kill bacteria coating the smaller bits.

In this patient's case, the bullet hadn't fragmented at all but was firmly lodged in his skull. The residents had decided it was more dangerous to take it out than to leave it in. So they sewed up the skin over it and treated him with antibiotics, keeping the patient in the hospital to monitor his wound for signs of infection. Despite the antibiotics, when Glick removed the man's bandage and pressed down lightly on the wound, a bit of fluid—possibly pus—appeared.

If the wound had been anywhere but the patient's head, such a small and ambiguous sign might not have been cause for alarm; it would probably have meant a change in his antibiotics and some watchful waiting to see if the drugs and his natural defenses could clear the infection. But a brain abscess, unlike a pimple, a boil, or even an infected surgical site on a limb, is a serious medical emergency. This is true for two reasons.

First, the brain is immunologically privileged, meaning the normal weapons the body uses to fight infection can't easily gain access to it. This sequestration is accomplished by what is known as the blood-brain barrier. As in the rest of the body, the brain's arteries branch into smaller vessels called arterioles and then into capillaries. In most of the body, these capillaries are relatively leaky, meaning many different molecules and cells can make it through their walls, either by diffusion or, in the case of white blood cells—which do most of the work in protecting us from bacterial infection—by diapedesis, a kind of scooching through gaps in the vessel walls.

The ease with which many substances can pass through the walls of capillaries has been known for over a hundred years. So in 1885, when the German bacteriologist Paul Ehrlich noticed that a blue dye injected into a mouse's arteries stained every tissue in its body except its brain, he wasn't surprised that the dye leaked out of the animal's vessels to stain its muscles and other organs, but only that it hadn't stained the mouse's brain. At the time, he assumed it was because the brain tissue was inherently less stainable by the dye. It wasn't until around 1906, when Ehrlich and his student Edwin Goldman thought to inject the dye directly into the brain, with the result that only the brain and no other tissue was stained, that the concept of a highly selective screen between the brain and the rest of the body was born.

We now know that capillaries in the brain are generally less leaky than capillaries elsewhere and for the most part don't have the gaps found in other capillaries that allow white blood cells through. This extra security keeps the brain in a strictly regulated environment, protecting it from many substances circulating in the rest of the body. There are some compounds that can make it through—MSG, caffeine, Bud Light—but for the most part an intact blood-brain barrier keeps the brain safe, both from toxins and from bacteria and viruses. Until recently, it was believed that if a bacterium or virus did get through the barrier, it couldn't be wiped out by the body's normal housekeepers—that the immune cells involved in mopping up unwanted microbes simply couldn't make it through. It has recently been shown that this is an oversimplification and that there are white blood cells in many parts of the brain, but no one is quite sure which parts and how many. What is certain is that the blood-brain barrier makes it hard to design drugs that can make it into the brain to help those cells cure an infection.

The second reason a brain abscess requires immediate surgery is the simple fact of the skull. If allowed to develop unchecked, a tiny colony of bacteria can rapidly grow in the brain (some colonies may double in size every half hour), while attracting any white blood cells able to reach the site. In an attempt to fight the bacteria, those white blood cells wreak a kind of destruction on nearby brain cells that is known as liquefactive necrosis. Meanwhile, the bacteria continue multiplying, the white blood cells send out messages recruiting other white blood cells, and the whole mess enlarges until the collection of bacteria, cells, and cell debris begins to push the brain out of the way. Because it's encased in the skull, there isn't anywhere for the brain to go. It will be compressed against the inside of the skull until the pressure becomes so great that the brain starts dribbling down toward the foramen magnum, the hole where the spinal cord leaves the skull. Once that happens, if surgery to drain the infection isn't performed within an hour or two, the patient will die, as the pressure on the brain stem prevents it from regulating breathing and heart rate.

That was why Glick and Song would be operating that evening on the man with the bullet in his head, although they didn't explain it to the patient in such detail: in less than thirty seconds, Glick had looked at the wound, found out when he'd eaten last (9:00 p.m. two nights before), and told him they would take him to the OR later that day. Then she was out the door and headed to the pediatric ward with Song at her side. As they walked, he peered over her shoulder, watching her sketch on a scrap of paper a couple of lines representing the type and location of incision she wanted to use when removing the bullet.

IT IS THAT INCISION I see in front of me now, in the OR. With Glick in the operating room, Song can proceed to what the two consider to be the start of the real operation: the craniotomy, in which they'll open the man's skull. That the bullet hasn't completely penetrated the skull is good news, but how much damage was done to the brain and blood vessels on the other side of the bone is unclear. Many areas of cortex can be damaged (if the damage covers a small area) without any effect on a person's ability to function, and this man had shown no signs of brain damage. But if the bullet had nicked a vessel and was itself serving as a plug for the hole it had created, extracting it without first gaining enough access to the brain to repair the vessel could cause a life-threatening bleed, which is why Glick compared removing the bullet to pulling a finger out of a dam.

Now, as she looks on, Song is preparing to gain that access; he picks up a power tool known as a perforator and prepares to drill a hole in the patient's skull. I imagine the man's brain on the other side of the bone, just millimeters from the tip of Song's drill. Immediately surrounding his brain will be a thin, clingy, whitish wrapping, the organic equivalent of tissue paper, called the pia mater. This wrapping covers the brain so closely, following the contours of each sulcus (groove) and gyrus (ridge) of the cerebral hemispheres, that the pia itself is scarcely visible. Around the pia mater is the arachnoid, another soft, moist covering, named for its resemblance to a spiderweb. Between these two layers is a thin layer of cerebrospinal fluid.

Cerebrospinal fluid (CSF) is produced in the ventricles, open spaces deep inside the brain that remained as it developed from the neural tube.

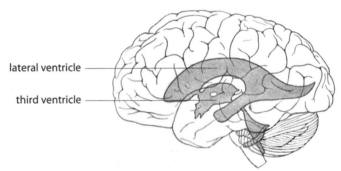

lateral ventricle ⸺⸺⸺⸺

third ventricle ⸺⸺⸺⸺

After its production, the CSF trickles out of the ventricles and down around the spinal cord, then is pushed back up around the outside of the brain by the arrival of more CSF.

The CSF keeps the brain floating inside your head. As the brain is about 80 percent water, it is both fragile and heavy; the CSF decreases its effective weight from over three pounds—which is what it would be just sitting on a table, where, like soft Jell-O, its own weight might tear it—to just under two ounces, allowing it to stay plump and preventing its collapse onto the floor of your skull.

Around the arachnoid runs the dura mater, a rough, fibrous layer like a tarpaulin. Unlike the arachnoid, the pia mater, and the brain itself, the dura is pain sensitive, and some researchers theorize that certain kinds of headaches are due to irritation or stretching of the dura.

The dura is located right up against the inside of the skull and has several long channels in it called sinuses. These sinuses serve as veins, draining used blood from the brain; the CSF is also dumped into them after it has made its trip around the brain and spinal cord. The largest of these channels in the dura, the superior sagittal sinus, runs the length of the head just under the skull—from the forehead, up over the top of the brain, to the base of the skull at the back of the head.

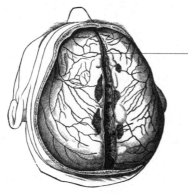

superior sagittal sinus

Around the dura is the skull—the box that keeps its valuable contents safe. Now imagine being a neurosurgeon. You are presented with this bony box, gift wrapped in two layers of connective tissue, a layer of fat and a layer of skin decorated with thickly placed hairs. Imagine you know there's a life-threatening problem inside that box—an artery with a weak spot ballooning out to form an aneurysm that could burst and cause a stroke, a tumor or abscess growing and compressing the brain. How do you get inside that box to save your patient? Shaving the hair and peeling away the skin and connective tissue will be relatively easy, if you can find a way to keep the superficial arteries in the scalp—of which there are many—from bleeding so much you can't see what you're doing. But now what? There you are, staring at the slick white surface of bone through the wide red lips of the wound you've made, knowing that just inside, right up against the wall of that box, is the very self of your patient, embodied in a structure as destructible as a custard. Any instrument you use to break through the thickness of the skull, any amount of force you apply to it to gain entry, may—if it goes just half a centimeter too far—wreak havoc on the person you are trying to save.

Even in ancient times, people did figure out a way to safely breach the skull of a living person. A number of prehistoric human skulls show evidence that holes had been made in them while their owners were still alive. While no one knows exactly why they were made, there are several ways anthropologists think these trephinations, as they're called, were performed. Some appear to have been made simply by scraping repeatedly at an area of the skull with a shell or sharpened rock until enough bone was removed to expose the dura. Another method apparently involved making a series of four intersecting cuts in the skull, like a tic-tac-toe board, with the center square of bone then surrounded by the deepest parts of each cut so that it could be easily removed. There is also evidence that in ancient times the skull may have been breached by drilling a series of holes with a hand drill, outlining in perforations the piece of bone to be removed. This method is still in use today in certain circumstances; indeed, Glick and Song are using a variation on it to remove the bullet from their patient's skull.

The development of power tools made penetrating the skull easier, although it brought with it the danger of driving those tools, still spinning, into the brain. Harvey Cushing, an early-twentieth-century surgeon generally known as the father of neurosurgery in this country, distrusted power tools, still new at the end of his career, as he thought it too easy to lose control of them. Such concerns remain. While modern drills are made with clutch-release mechanisms so that they stop automatically once the bone has been penetrated and resistance to the drill drops, they have been known to malfunction and be driven into a patient's brain. Now, as Song positions the per-

forator for his first burr hole, I hear Glick say to him, "Don't plunge—
if you plunge here, it's bad."

While Song pushes the spinning perforator into a spot in the patient's skull just above the bullet, the scrub nurse leans down and uses
what looks like a turkey baster to drip sterile saline solution into the
wound. The saline washes away blood and bone dust in a steady,
mucky stream and also keeps the cutting blade cool; overheating
could cause the perforator to seize up or, worse, to fry the brain once
through the skull. When he's done, Song has made a perfectly round
hole about a centimeter in diameter. Glick puts the tip of her suction
tool at the edge of the hole, and blood comes slipping out in a twist
of red through the clear plastic tubing attached to the vacuum pump.

Song makes two more holes, and then Glick says, "Now, just bite
as you go." The nurse hands Song a pair of Kerrison rongeurs, which
look like a delicate set of pliers, but with a right-angled grip like a
gun. He uses them to pull away little pieces of the man's skull, joining the holes to create a larger opening above and around the sides
of the bullet.

Song grunts as he pries off a bit of bone. Neurosurgery, famous
for its practitioners' delicacy and attention to detail, also requires a fair
amount of brute strength. Song's task at the moment is so strenuous
that Glick says she lifted weights during her own residency just to stay
equal to it. He grunts again. "Don't I sound like ortho?" he asks, a jok-
ing reference to orthopedic surgeons, whose job requires the same
kind of strength but who are sometimes, unfairly, viewed in medical
circles as the opposite of neurosurgeons: crude, brute-strength types,
lacking in finesse and intellectual prowess.

At this moment, Song's and Glick's hands are moving within a
space the size of a shoe box, manipulating instruments working in an
area the size of a half-dollar. Both sets of hands move continuously at
lightning speed, even as their conversation proceeds at a normal pace.
It's uncanny, like the Hans Christian Andersen fairy tale of the red

shoes that forced their owner's feet to keep on dancing, whatever else she might be doing at the same time. In a matter of minutes, Song removes an arc of bone from above and around the sides of the bullet.

"See, there's the healthy dura," Glick says. And that's why I wanted to go lateral, 'cause over here is dangerous. She's pointing to a spot, still covered with skin, below the bullet. I now realize that although I had imagined the patient before us lying on his back, with the crown of his head facing us, the truth is that under all the drapes he is lying on his side, facing to our right. Between the bullet and the ceiling is his left ear, and between the bullet and the floor is his right ear. The crescent of bone Song has removed sits like a letter *C* cupping the bullet, lying between it and the patient's left ear, while the skin-covered spot Glick wanted to avoid is close to the midline of the patient's head. "Mike wanted to go over here," Glick says to me, pointing again to the skin-covered spot at the midline, "'cause Mike loves danger."

I ought to know what danger she's talking about, but I've been up and with her since before sunrise. It's over ninety degrees in the operating room, and I'm sweating through the synthetic scrubs and bouffant cap I'm wearing, and wondering, for the second time in my life, if I might be in danger of passing out. (The first time was only days before, as I watched Glick place a tube in the brain of a tiny infant.) I'm holding a notebook in which I'm supposed to be taking notes, but I've forgotten all of that, along with the anatomy I'm supposed to know. I've forgotten everything except the two sets of hands and the wound in front of me.

EARLIER, AFTER GLICK had told the man with the bullet in his head they'd be operating on him later, she and Song went to check on a baby girl whom Glick had treated for a hemorrhagic stroke.

There are two broad categories of stroke: ischemic and hemorrhagic. An ischemic stroke is often due to an embolus — a bit of material, usually a blood clot but sometimes a bubble of air or a bit of fat—that floats through the bloodstream until it arrives at an artery in the brain too small to let it pass. The embolus lodges there, blocking blood flow. A hemorrhagic stroke occurs when a weakness or malformation in an artery causes it to burst, flooding the brain with blood and, like a burst water main, cutting off the supply to areas downstream. Either way, the result is usually disastrous and often fatal, a large-scale killing off of brain cells by suffocation. In the case of hemorrhagic stroke, the picture is complicated by the fact that the heart continues to pump blood into the brain, where it pools and compresses the brain against the skull. It's important to drain the blood as soon as possible, for the same reason that it's important to drain an abscess.

Why this baby had had a stroke remained a mystery; although hemorrhagic strokes in infants can be linked to cocaine use by the mother while pregnant (a frequent concern at Cook County), this baby's mother appeared clean. Glick was on call when the baby was rushed to the hospital, so she had been the one to drain the blood from her brain. She had begun the surgery around 9:00 p.m., she said, after a typically packed day, and was already worried. "We were operating in a really tired state," she said.

I later spoke with one of Glick's longtime friends. "Can you imagine having someone's brain open in front of you and being sleepy?" the friend—an artist, teacher, and extremely energetic woman herself— asked. "She must have such incredible energy reserves."

And in fact, that's how Glick describes what she relies on in such situations. "You have to get all your energy focused into, like, one little point," she told me. "You ever hear Michael Jordan talk about playing basketball, how he gets in the zone? Well, that's how it feels sometimes when you do an operation." It's as if "you have this reserve and you kind of delve into it," she said. "Like when I was pregnant— I was eight or nine months pregnant, and I'd have to get up at three in the morning to do an operation and I'd be like, 'Oh, my God, what is this going to do to my baby? I'm going to be on my feet in the middle of the night!' So I'd just calm myself down and say, 'Ok, kid, your mom's a neurosurgeon. We're going to do surgery; we're going to save a life here.'" And while she does regularly have to operate when she's tired, Glick says she has a strategy. "When you're tired, you're more likely to make mistakes. So when I'm tired, I just try and do simple, basic things that I know how to do—I won't try anything new."

So presumably that was her mind-set when she began operating on the baby with the stroke. But even without trying anything new, unexpected situations arise, and in this case, disaster struck: the artery in the infant's brain began to bleed again during the operation, copiously. "The baby was exsanguinating on the table and nearly died—I nearly lost her," Glick said. "It was really almost uncontrollable. And then at some point, the baby's heart stopped. And I was like, 'Stay calm, everybody stay cool.' You know, some people get all crazy, are throwing stuff around and yelling and swearing, but I just have to stay calm."

How she accomplishes that is through a sort of spiritual mishmosh that she's accumulated from travel, Judaism, and a voracious reading habit. It was on a medical tour of China in 1978, shortly after the country opened its borders to Americans, that Glick was introduced to tai chi. "I went out one morning at, like, seven a.m., and everyone—thousands of people were out in the streets doing tai chi. It was like something out of a painting—you know, this purple sky with all these pagodas. And there were these four people doing tai chi against the sunrise, and they waved me over and I did tai chi with them." On that trip she bought a pair of the soft-soled shoes traditionally worn for tai chi, a pair she still wears for her daily practice, which she says helps keep her "on the path," a phrase she uses to refer, at various times, to neurosurgery, to life itself, or to spirituality and Judaism in particular.

In addition to her private study of Judaism, Glick is an active member of a Jewish spiritual group. Known as Lomdim, which means "scholar" or "study," the group has about forty members, who form a close-knit association of "writers, artists, lawyers, doctors—a lot of doctors," she says. The members have banded together to hold weekly services followed by a potluck lunch, and serve almost as an extended family for her. "Two people met in the group, so now we've had a marriage, births, deaths," she told me with obvious pride.

"It's funny," Glick said to me once. "You don't think of your neurosurgeon as the spiritual, uplifting one." The stereotype of surgeons in general and neurosurgeons in particular is that they are more interested in the mechanics of the human body than in the spirit that makes it human. But Glick says she uses spirituality in her daily practice as a neurosurgeon, giving the example of her hectic Friday-morning clinic, where she sees pre- and post-op patients in an outpatient setting. "There's supposed to be forty patients, forty-five, but there's like sixty. The patients all get there at the same time and get numbers from one to sixty. It's like you try to do a good job, be good to your patients, but it's impossible. So I was just losing it all the time. And then Thursday nights I started reading something—Torah or something—something that puts me in the right mind-set, and I'll tell you something, it's changed my life."

That reading is in addition to her regular reading, which is perpetual and varied. "I'm always reading something on parenting or spirituality, some literature book, a goofball book." (Two examples of goofball books would be *Surfing Rabbi*, Rabbi Nachum Shifren's autobiographical account of his transition from a secular assimilated Jewish Malibu surfer to a devoutly orthodox Jewish Malibu surfer, and *Driving Mr. Albert*, Michael Paterniti's book about traveling across the country with the pathologist who performed the autopsy on and then absconded with Einstein's brain, both of which she was reading during the time I spent with her.) "And then there's the book-club book," which at that time was, at her suggestion, *One Hundred Years of Solitude.* She'd lately also begun to read William Blake. "I just recently got into poetry. I never really was before—I found poetry intimidating. Neurosurgery wasn't intimidating, but poetry!"

When we arrived at her bedside, the baby looked like a tiny maharaja, turbaned in bandages and covered with a blanket printed with elephants and teddy bears. She was silent and still, kept in a coma by the administration of barbiturates, which Glick hoped would keep her brain from swelling after the irritation caused by the stroke and then the surgery. The baby's mother, who looked about twenty years old, sat beside the crib, reading a Harry Potter book. When Glick walked in, the woman immediately put her finger in the book and looked up; there was exhaustion in her eyes, and behind them something strangely empty that must have been shock, but over it all was a hyperalert attention to anything Glick said.

Glick explained quickly that she wanted to delay getting a follow-up CT scan in an attempt to give the baby time to heal as much as possible before moving her, but that because they needed to see how the baby's brain was doing, they would get one the next day, which was as long as Glick felt she could wait. As Glick left, she said to Song, "When they do the scan, everybody goes," meaning both the medical and the surgical teams responsible for the baby's care should go along, in case moving the baby caused her to start bleeding again, which would require emergency surgery.

Then it was time for Glick to leave for services at Lomdim. In the car on the way back to Evanston to pick up her kids, she said, "Anyway, the baby's still alive. It's amazing." Which was true but left out a lot of the quality-of-life issues she had been talking about on the drive in: whether the baby would have permanent brain damage, if she could develop normally, what her daily life would be like. As we drove past strip malls and through low-slung green suburbia, I asked Glick if she thought the baby would be OK. She shook her head. "I mean,

I think there's a chance, but—" Then she said, "These stories, each one is more tragic than the next. Isn't it just heartbreaking to see that baby, and then the man shot, and the tumors? I don't think my other friends really know what I do all day. I mean, all these images— uh-oh."

She'd been cut off by the sound of her beeper, but it was only her husband, Terry. Terry is an endocrinologist and works in a hospital just a block away from Cook County. In addition to his job, Terry coaches a boys' soccer team, which meant he wouldn't be able to come to services that day. Glick called him from her cell phone and asked him to have the kids ready and on the porch when we got to their house.

They were. Or at least Jonah, her four-year-old, was, sitting next to Terry on the glider that takes up a good third of their front porch. The porch is the only small thing about their house, although its clutter is in harmony with the house's interior. The glider sits against a railing on which is balanced an enormous rural-style mailbox, beside several plants and some bubble-blowing paraphernalia, and under a string of Tibetan prayer flags hung from a pillar still wrapped, in August, with sheets of cellophane printed with googly eyes from some previous Halloween. "We never take anything down from the holidays," Glick told me cheerfully on a previous visit, as I walked past a permanently installed HAPPY HANUKKAH sign made by one of her boys. That sign hangs at the doorway to the living room, in which every available space is covered with toys, hung with art, stacked with books, or decorated with plants. Toward the back of the house is the stairway to the basement. That stairway's wall is hung with more of her sons' work and is known within the family as the Gallery. Beyond the Gallery is the kitchen, lined with wooden cabinets that Glick ordered from a laboratory-supply company and that anyone who has ever done research in a wet lab would recognize. The kitchen is tiled with tiny multicolored hexagonal tiles that Glick chose because, she says, she wanted the room to look like an Italian restaurant. Near the window are two parakeets, one blue and the other green, named Blueberry and Spinach by Daniel, nine, who came running out of the house as we pulled up.

Not stopping to join his brother, who trailed after him, Daniel raced down the porch steps and kept running until he reached the car, at which point he climbed onto its roof. Glick hauled him down, looked at his finger, asked him to bend it, handed him a yarmulke, wiped chocolate off Jonah's face, made sure he had a diaper and a clean shirt, and loaded them into the car, waving good-bye to Terry.

That Glick, at a time in her life when many women would be e-mailing their children at college, is still finishing up the potty training of her youngest son is testimony to the difficulties of being a woman in neurosurgery. "When I was board certified, I was like the twenty-second woman out of four thousand men," she told me. Things haven't changed much since then; in 2004, there were about 3,250 certified and practicing neurosurgeons. Of them, only 122 were women.

Why there aren't more is a question with a few clear answers and a couple of muddier ones. Surgery in general, and neurosurgery especially, requires years of arduous training. Most medical-school graduates are around twenty-six years old; after graduation, they go on to a residency, which in the case of neurosurgery lasts for six or seven years. During that time, until recently, a neurosurgical resident could expect to spend between 80 and 130 hours a week in the hospital, which meant that in order to become a neurosurgeon, a woman had to devote essentially every waking minute of all of her prime childbearing years to the goal.* Once that goal is reached, a new neuro-

---

* In 2003, the Accreditation Council for Graduate Medical Education, the accrediting body for teaching hospitals, mandated that residents work no more than 80 hours per week. It remains to be seen whether this policy will stand. Already many neurosurgical residency programs have petitioned for and received permission to increase their residents' hours to an average of 88 hours on duty per week.

surgeon still must make a name for herself in a career in which taking time off is looked down on not only for social but also for practical reasons: it behooves a surgeon to stay in practice, as each case requires a level of mental and physical dexterity that comes only from repeated and recent experience.

In light of all this, it's easy to understand a colleague Glick encountered at a meeting of a group called Women in Neurosurgery. Glick had suggested that issues the group might discuss could include ways of balancing a career and a family. "And this woman," she told me, "turns to me and goes, in this nasty voice, 'When you entered neurosurgery, you entered the convent. You'd better get that through your head.'"

Yet the society in which Glick found herself upon completing medical school was hardly one of cloistered femininity. One of her fellow residents (so this would have been around 1980) said to her, in explaining why he didn't think women should be neurosurgeons, "If God wanted women to fly, he would have made the sky pink." Then there was her graduation party, which was combined with a celebration honoring a departing attending physician. "They invited every resident my attending had ever trained, so it was like a hundred guys and me," she told me. "They're making toasts and there's desserts and cigars and wine, and then somebody turns on some music, and a stripper gets on the table."

Today things have gotten better for women in neurosurgery, a change that has come about because of women like Glick, and especially because of one particular woman, the neurosurgeon Frances Conley. "There's like AC and BC—After Conley and Before Conley," Glick says. Conley was, until her recent retirement, a practicing neurosurgeon at Stanford University. Right around the time Anita Hill was detailing for Congress her allegations of Clarence Thomas's inappropriate behavior toward her, Conley wrote a letter to the *San Francisco Chronicle* describing her experiences of gender discrimination within neurosurgery, experiences remarkably similar to Glick's.

The article made an enormous stir, partly because there were— and still are—those who questioned Conley's motives, as well as her method of naming, in a public forum and without formal charges, the men she saw as guilty of discrimination. Nonetheless, Conley's letter and subsequent book, *Walking Out on the Boys,* served as a spotlight that, aided by the lens of the Hill-Thomas case and American society's growing awareness of gender discrimination in the workplace, served to dampen the macho culture within neurosurgery.

Conley herself was married but opted not to have children; Glick waited until she was almost forty and had been appointed associate professor before having her first. "Geriatric motherhood," she called it, when we ran into a friend of hers on the street whose grandson is a playmate of Jonah's. "I'm writing a book on women who are having kids over forty," she said, "called *From Maternity to Menopause—in Ten Days.*"

Although she jokes about it, Daniel's birth caused her something of a crisis. Glick told me that at the end of what sounded like a particularly arduous and complicated labor, she looked at her newborn son and said, "OK, I'm not going back to work, and his name is Daniel, which means 'God is my judge.'"

Although she did go back to work, Glick now officially takes Mondays off, which makes her something of a trailblazer, as there aren't many part-time neurosurgeons. "I've kind of decelerated my career so I can be with my kids in the early years," she says. "But you have to be careful, because you can be relegated to the sort of 'mommy track.'" In order to avoid that fate, Glick says she's learned to toot her own horn a bit. On the first day I met her, she told me that she was on the board of the journal *Neurosurgery.* "Can you pick me out?" she asked, pointing to a group picture of the board hanging in her office. Of course I could: it showed about two dozen gray-suited men and Glick, who was the first woman ever appointed to the board, an honor she received because she asked for it, after she'd spent ten years as a peer reviewer for the journal.

That she had to ask, and that her request was immediately granted, is an illustration of the kind of discrimination Glick thinks is predominant in neurosurgery today, which she calls "discrimination by neglect." "They're just not thinking of you at all," she says. And while there is still something of a gender clash within neurosurgery, its ramifications seem more benign today. "It's interesting," Glick says, "talking about men and women. I'll say to the residents, 'OK, go through the operation step-by-step beforehand so it'll be like a well-choreographed dance.' And the residents — men — will sometimes say to me, 'No, it's more like a football game.'"

It is this history of discrimination, difficult choices, and changing culture that is behind the glee Glick has in telling one of her favorite stories about Daniel, now sitting with Jonah in the backseat as we drive to temple. According to Glick, when Daniel was three years old, he was asked by a well-meaning adult if he was going to be a neuro-surgeon when he grew up, to which he responded, disdainfully, "*Girls* are neurosurgeons. *Boys* are endocrinologists."

IN THE OR, Glick says to me over her shoulder, "He wants to take that bullet out so bad." Song has been working at their patient's skull for about ten minutes, pulling away bits of it until there is no longer any bone surrounding the bullet, which is just barely lodged in the dura covering the pink brain matter itself. The bullet sits there like a loose tooth, clearly ready to come out at the slightest touch.

"When you take it out," Song says, without looking up, "you have to have a big metal bowl and you have to drop it in there with a clunk."

"That's part of the drama," Glick adds.

At this point she is dribbling saline solution in the surgical field, and the stream of liquid knocks the bullet out of the wound. There is no rush of blood to follow it. It seems as if there ought to be a mo-ment of surprise, or even laughter, but without missing a beat Song retrieves the bullet with his forceps and calls, "Bowl!" The nurse holds out a stainless-steel bowl, and he tosses the bullet in. It lands almost silently. "Hey, that didn't make the right sound," he says, and reaches into the bowl with the forceps. He picks up the bullet and flings it back into the bowl. This time it makes a slight *thuck* but bounces out of the bowl, falling amid the folds of paper and plastic drapes arranged beneath the patient's head to catch the blood and saline solution dripping from the wound. Song grabs the bullet again and throws it into the bowl a third time, where it lands with a muffled thump. "Defective bowl," he mutters as he gets back to work, pulling a few more bits of bone from the wound.

THE DRIVE TO THE temple was long enough that the boys were antsy; when Glick parked the car, they exploded out of it and ran yowling in and out of the hedge surrounding the building. "Daniel— this is a temple! This is a temple!" Glick called after them. It seemed OK, though, and also OK that when they got inside the temple's library, an intimate room filled with folding chairs, the service was already well under way. Lomdim is the type of group where if the members are having trouble with a song, they may stop in the middle of it to have a discussion about the best key and the right pacing, during which someone might pipe up, "And what are the words again?" Glick took her shoes off almost as soon as she sat down, and throughout much of the service she whispered to me, explaining Jewish traditions, pointing out members of the group whom she thought I'd find interesting because they were either doctors or writers, showing me her favorite prayers in the prayer book.

Science and religion are intertwined in Glick's mind. "I think science answers how and spirituality answers why," she says. "I'm not in that field of medicine of 'Where is the mind?' or 'Where is the soul?'" she says, preferring to use her religion to explore such questions. And yet when she gives me her definitions of God and religion, her work crops up. "What is God? Is it nature, is it music, is it beauty? I think it's all those things," she told me. "How you feel in life when you see the *Mona Lisa*, hear Glenn Gould playing the *Goldberg Variations*, or when you see a great neurosurgical operation—I think this is God's work. I think believing in God means that you think what you do has meaning beyond just yourself, that your actions have greater meaning than just you."

One might expect that Glick would use her religion to ponder what happens to her patients who die. Like all neurosurgeons who specialize in brain tumors, Glick tends to measure postoperative survival in months: one of her most triumphant stories involves a surgery she performed on a young mother with a brain tumor. Glick's colleagues had deemed the woman beyond help, but Glick operated anyway. When the patient died nine months later, Glick's associates agreed that the surgery had been worth it—they'd all operated in hope of giving a patient less time than that. But while her job entails functioning in a milieu of what she calls "this in-your-face mortality," Glick says she doesn't spend any time wondering what happens to her patients after death. "I see people die every week, but I don't think about what happens after death," she said. "I have no opinions on it. Worry about what happens when you're alive."

After the service, Glick collected Daniel and Jonah and took them back home, where she and Terry were hosting a potluck for the Lomdim group. Afterward, when the guests began to disperse, Glick headed back to the hospital to supervise Song as he removed the bullet from the head of the man we'd met that morning. As we drove south along Lake Shore Drive for the second time that day, she called him on her cell phone and told him not to start without her.

SONG'S PAPER SHOE covers have fallen halfway off his feet, dragged down by the weight of the blood and saline solution they've soaked up from the floor. He's drilling small holes in the patient's skull to anchor the sutures he'll use to close the dura. Meanwhile, Glick puts some bone wax to soak in a solution of bacitracin. The bone wax will cover the spot where Song has removed a portion of the patient's skull—which will never grow back—and the bacitracin will help kill any remaining bacteria. In a gesture signaling the end of the neurosurgical part of the operation, one of the nurses brings Song a stool to sit on, twirls it to the right height, and mops up the puddle he's standing in. The wound in the patient's head now looks neat and tidy, if such a thing is possible: its edges are clean, there are no stray bits of tissue, the bleeding has slowed.

"See, it's a little operation," Glick says, "but if you lose control—it's like the other day, with the baby and all that bleeding." A moment later she says, "OK, Dr. Song, I'm going to trust you," and steps away. We have been in the OR just under an hour. To me she says, "Is my thing, like, dripping wet?" indicating the sterile gown she has on over her scrubs. "I feel drenched." It's not, but surely the scrubs she's wearing underneath are, and her hair is now plastered to her head beneath her cap.

As we leave, she says, "I always use the KISS technique. You know what that is? Keep It Simple, Stupid. Instead of going looking for the superior sagittal sinus and controlling it, just don't see it." Finally I understand the danger she's been alluding to and her discussion with Song about where to make the incision. The bullet entered the man's head just beside the superior sagittal sinus, that venous channel in the dura running along his head.

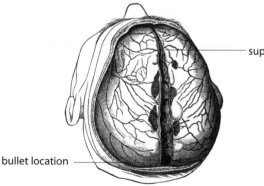

superior sagittal sinus

bullet location

Had the bullet hit him just a centimeter closer to the midline of his head, it would have penetrated the sinus, in which case the man might have died of blood loss before reaching the hospital. The incision Glick directed Song to use allowed them to completely bypass the vessel, thus avoiding the possibility of causing the same problem themselves.

"Wasn't that interesting, though? Seeing that bullet stuck in that guy's head?" Glick asks back in her office. As she gets ready to leave, she calls Terry, who tells her he's rented *The Pledge* with Jack Nicholson to watch that night. But she's not interested. "Oh, no, that's too creepy," she says into the phone. Then to me, "I've heard it has a really disturbing ending. Who needs that? I want something light. Maybe I'll just go watch *Barney*."

On our way out, apropos of nothing, Glick says, "You know, people get falsely impressed when you tell them you're a neurosurgeon, like, 'Oh, wow, you must be brilliant.' I'd rather be anonymous." Once we're in the car, she says, "Oh, I didn't get to spend much time with my boys today." Then the sky opens over us as we leave the parking garage. "Look how clear it is tonight!" she cries as we drive north toward Chicago's downtown, the Sears Tower dark against a sky streaked with amber and purple.

Tomorrow the baby with the stroke will have a CT scan, which will show no signs of rebleeding. And the day after that, Glick and Song will be standing in her office when the door opens to admit the man they've just finished operating on. He'll be dressed in a hospital gown, his head covered with a little gauze cap, but he'll be walking on his own. Song will remove the cap and take a look at the wound. "Looks perfect," he'll say.

"Well, we never say 'perfect,'" Glick will answer, "but it looks good."

Now Glick comes back to the baby again, as if she's been thinking about my question earlier in the day. The stroke has severely damaged most of the right side of the baby's brain, but that still leaves the left side. "So maybe the left could be dominant," she says. "It's really interesting, in children before the age of speech and writing, you can do, like, hemispherectomies"— meaning removal of half the brain— "and the baby will be OK."

Something about Glick's day—the gunshot wound, the baby, and the miraculous possibility of recovery—reminds me of a prayer Glick showed me in Lomdim's prayer book. It is known as the blessing of Asher Yatzar and goes like this:

> Praised are You, Lord our God, King of the universe who with wisdom fashioned the human body, creating openings, arteries, glands and organs, marvelous in structure, intricate in design. Should but one of them, by being blocked or opened, fail to function, it would be impossible to exist. Praised are You, Lord, healer of all flesh who sustains our bodies in wondrous ways.

Conception	6 weeks	10 weeks	30 weeks	6 years	Adolescence	Adulthood	Old Age	Death

Birth

When your neural tube first developed, it was made of a single sheet of cells. Soon, though—about six weeks after you were conceived—those cells, known as neural progenitor cells, began to divide, producing neurons. Early on, those divisions were so fast that the number of cells in your embryonic cerebral cortex more than doubled each day.

Most of the cell divisions occurred on the inside surface of the neural tube, the surface that would later become the wall of the ventricles where CSF is produced, deep inside the brain. Once a cell had divided and produced a neuron, however, that neuron migrated to the outer surface of your neural tube, toward what would become the outer surface of your brain.

As more neurons were born and traveled outward, they were forced to squeeze through the thicket of cells already generated. To help them on their way, some cells, rather than becoming neurons, became radial glia. These cells stretched long, thin processes from the inside to the outside surface of your neural tube. Throughout your brain's development, the radial glia clung with one process to the inner ventricular surface, and with the other, to the outer surface of your growing brain, stretching as your cortex thickened, allowing each round of newly minted neurons to use them as guide ropes to help in their outward voyage.

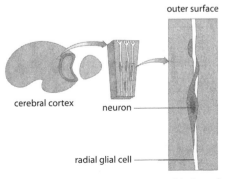

outer surface

cerebral cortex

neuron

radial glial cell

ventricular surface

Developmental biologists are beginning to show that even in your very early neural tube, the migrating neurons already knew what they were going to be when they grew up. The adult human cortex is made up of more than fifty separate functional areas, each responsible for some part of our capacities. The borders between those areas are, like borders between nations, often invisible and independent of geographic boundaries. There are no apparent physical or organizational differences between the neurons in one functional area and those in another. Each is apparently formed simply by the unification of their populations of neurons for a common cause. The cells in the part of our cortex where we recognize human faces (known as the fusiform face area and located in the fusiform gyrus, itself located on the underside of the temporal lobe) look just like those in the motor cortex, involved in the planning and execution of movements. Nevertheless, most of us seem to use that one particular little spot in our fusiform gyri to recognize Aunt Lulabelle, and use our motor cortex to initiate the movements required to crack our knuckles.

It is now being shown that those functional areas of cortex were already being mapped out at the neural tube stage, and that soon after each neuron was born, its fate was largely decided. Apparently, at that time, some newborn neurons become "organizers," releasing proteins called morphogens. As those proteins diffused outward, they set up a concentration gradient, with more of a morphogen close to the cell releasing it and less of it farther away. Two organizers, by secreting two different morphogens, can thus set up a sort of Cartesian coordinate map, with every point between them having a unique combination of concentrations of the two proteins.

The theory is that an emigrating neuron plowing through those gradients on its way to the surface of the brain will reach a spot uniquely labeled by its particular concentrations of morphogens. That particular combination induces the emigrating neuron to turn some of its own genes off and turn others on, causing it to develop into a particular type of neuron, appropriate for the area in which it finds itself.

This type of signaling based on gradients of diffusible molecules is similar to the molecular signaling that ensures that, whether we are tall or short, black or white, male or female, we (for the most part) are each born with two arms and two legs, with those limbs located in approximately the same place relative to our shoulders, heads, and feet. In fact, our motor cortices are arranged in a similar fashion, with a standardized map of our bodies contained within them. For instance, in your motor cortex, the neurons that tell your foot to move are tucked in at the top of your brain, between the two hemispheres, and the neurons governing your tongue are located at the side of your brain. That somatotopic map in your brain was represented by the neurosurgeon Wilder Penfield like this:

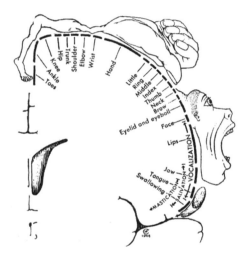

Reproduced from Penfield and Rasmussen, The Cerebral Cortex of Man, *1950, published with permission of the Curator, the Wilder Penfield Archive, Montreal Neurological Institute.*

This is a coronal section, meaning it's the view people would get of your brain if, when you put on your headphones, they sliced off the front half of your head. In this case, it's just the left half of that slice.

Because it's easy to tell whether and where someone is moving, it is well established that the motor cortex is necessary for movement, and that stimulating it results in movement. But we have other less quantifiable capacities, and it remains to be seen how much variation exists in the size, shape, and organization of functional areas of the brain, how such variation develops, and what it means. We know that, just as some are born with more prominent chins or longer fingers, some too are born with larger or smaller fusiform gyri. And just as some people are left handed and some are right handed, some of us recognize faces using our left fusiform gyri instead of the more commonly used right fusiform gyrus. But while we know that overall brain size doesn't correlate well with intelligence (Albert Einstein's weighed only 2.7 pounds, about 13 percent below average) and generally which part of the brain allows us to move our fingers, we don't yet know where in the brain a gift for physics or a love of piano playing arises. We may soon find out, however.

Check out these images of my brain. Cool, eh?

—CHRISTOF KOCH

2 | Watching the Brain

IN THE SUMMER OF 1998, Dr. John Gabrieli was in Boston, staying with his parents while helping his brother campaign for a Democratic congressional seat. The other members of the campaign were college students, at least twenty years younger than Gabrieli. "I think they viewed me as kind of pathetic," he later told me. "You know, doesn't have a job and he's working on the campaign and he's living with his parents," he said. "I don't really know, but I had this vague sense that they were all looking at me as this sort of sad person, just lucky to get a job for the summer."

That impression is, if inaccurate, maybe understandable. At well over six feet tall, Gabrieli has a slight stoop and a tight-jawed manner of speaking that, combined with his invariably self-deprecating sense of humor, keep him from ever appearing at ease. He dresses exclusively in khakis, button-downs, and either loafers or Hush Puppies. He wears brown tortoiseshell spectacles and combs his auburn hair smoothly from a side part. Comparisons to Clark Kent are made the more inevitable by his tendency to sprinkle his speech with exclamations worthy of Smallville (as in "Gee, I will say this, I feel like I had a happy childhood"), so it's not hard to picture his young co-workers quickly consigning him to their "loser" lists.

Imagine their surprise, then, when they turned on the radio at campaign headquarters and heard the host of the National Public Radio program *All Things Considered* announce his guest, a professor of psychology and neuroscience and an authority on memory: John Gabrieli of Stanford University.

Gabrieli had been invited to discuss the strange case of a man recently picked up by police in Jacksonville, Florida. Found wandering along the highway amid the smoke from a brush fire, the man had given his name as Terry Dibert, said he was twenty-three years old, and told the officers he needed to get back to Fort Bragg, North Carolina, where his army unit was stationed and his wife, Julie, was soon to give birth to their first child. Yet when the police called Fort Bragg, they learned that Dibert's unit had been gone for years.

Dibert was subsequently identified as a thirty-four-year-old accountant who'd been missing from his home — not in North Carolina but in central Pennsylvania — for over a week. He was, in fact, married to a woman named Julie, but she had borne the first of their three children eleven years earlier, while they were living at Fort Bragg. Dibert appeared to have lost the memories created during more than a decade of life, including those of his move to Pennsylvania, the birth of his children, and his new job as a business manager for a central Pennsylvania school district.

Such a phenomenon makes good headlines: a Web zine called *Paranormal Pages* came out with TIME TRAVELER GOES BACK TO 1987, as if that would, naturally, be the year anyone who could turn back the clock would visit. It soon became clear that Dibert wasn't claiming to have been abducted by space aliens, but that his condition had natural causes. At that point the legitimate press rushed to cover the story as well, which was why Gabrieli was featured on NPR.

In the course of the interview, Gabrieli explained that memories take years to "consolidate," a still poorly understood process of cementing them in the brain, and that if an injury occurs in the right spot at any point during those years, the memories still consolidating can be lost or temporarily inaccessible. He also touched on the theory of multiple memory systems, which explains why Dibert—whose injury was then still a mystery—could lose all memories of experiences from the previous eleven years yet still drive his car as proficiently as ever.

There was tension in Gabrieli's voice during the interview (he is, by his own account, extremely shy), and the segment lasted only a couple of minutes. Yet even this quick glimpse into his world gave his cocampaigners an image of him as an expert in a cutting-edge science, scouting ahead into the unknown territory of the mind.

Or at least, as employable. "Yeah," he told me, "later they all said, 'Were you on NPR? You have a job and everything?!'"

What Gabrieli has is more than a job. It is a quest that eats up the bulk of his waking hours ("Gee whiz, so let's see, most days I get in about seven a.m. and I leave about seven or eight p.m. Five days times twelve hours equals sixty, and most Saturdays and Sundays I'm in about half a day") and keeps him too busy for hobbies or even a lunch break. What Gabrieli has is a lab.

The Gab Lab, as it's called internally, is devoted to cognitive neuroscience, a field that scarcely existed thirty years ago but is today the subject of numerous international scientific meetings and dozens of journals. Cognitive neuroscience has been called the expensive branch of philosophy. It could also be called empiric philosophy: its practitioners try to figure out how and where we perform mental tasks or experience mental states.

When I first arrived at the lab, a catacomb of offices, conference rooms, and library space in one of the red-roofed sandstone buildings surrounding Stanford's mission-style quad, Gabrieli interrupted a meeting to introduce me around. As I followed him down the hall, I noticed an old *Peanuts* cartoon posted on the wall, a rueful nod to cognitive neuroscience's theoretical nature:

LINUS: When I grow up, I'd like to study about people. People interest me. I'd like to go to some big university and study all about people.

CHARLIE BROWN: I see . . .You want to learn about people so that with your knowledge you will be equipped to help them.

LINUS: No. I'm just nosy.

We reached a room in which two beautiful young women were seated side by side at computer monitors; one of them was Gabrieli's lab manager. She offered to find me a work space with a computer and then insisted when I told her not to bother, cheerfully installing me in an unused office. Everyone in the lab seemed young, happy, and eager; the bulletin boards were covered with postcards and photos of lab members on vacation in exotic places, and when I later spoke with some of them, it seemed none could praise Gabrieli enough, a fact he modestly brushes off. When I told him I had heard the word "flexible" over and over from colleagues when they described him, he said, "Well, if it means you don't know what you're doing and you have no particular mission and you just muddle through, then I think I'm flexible, sure."

While the scores of scientific papers Gabrieli has authored and the various national and international advisory boards on which he sits reveal that he clearly does know what he's doing, it would be hard to say Gabrieli has any one particular mission, as his interests are unusually eclectic. Cognitive neuroscience encompasses processes as varied as visual perception, mathematical calculations, and falling in love, so most cognitive neuroscientists specialize. Although Gabrieli's stated specialty is memory, he takes frequent side trips. His lab also investigates olfaction (the study of how we smell and what happens to our brain when we do), learning disorders (dyslexia, attention-deficit/hyperactivity disorder), face recognition, and, in a dabbling kind of way, the controversial question of how people of different races perceive one another visually.

But a common theme to most of the Gab Lab's work is a technique called functional magnetic resonance imaging, or fMRI. Functional MRI is one of the newest imaging tools used to study the brain. For decades, magnetic resonance imaging (MRI) has made possible high-definition images of soft-tissue structures that X-rays don't resolve well, like muscles, ligaments, and the brain. MRI was originally used to create static images, revolutionizing our ability to detect early cancers of organs like the liver or the kidney, as well as other soft-tissue abnormalities, such as torn ligaments, which are generally undetectable by X-ray. But in the early 1990s, scientists like Gabrieli began using magnetic resonance scanners to both show the architecture of the brain and watch it as it works—that is, as we think.

The basis of fMRI is a concept so simple most fifth-graders can rattle it off: blood provides working cells with oxygen and other nutrients and removes waste products like carbon dioxide. Because harder-working cells need more oxygen and nutrients and give off more waste, they need more blood. So if you could find some way to measure blood flow within the brain, you could theoretically determine when the brain—or a given part of it—is working hardest and when it is relatively quiescent.

This idea is not new. In his book *The Principles of Psychology*, William James, the nineteenth-century philosopher of mind, wrote of a contemporary, an Italian physician named Mosso. According to James, Mosso hypothesized that when we think, we must require increased blood flow to the brain. To prove his theory, he had human subjects lie on a table, which he then carefully balanced on a fulcrum. After instructing the subjects to remain absolutely motionless, he gave them various mental tasks. According to Mosso, as his subjects started thinking harder, the end of the table supporting their heads invariably sank slightly—a phenomenon he attributed to increased blood perfusing the brain tissue. While his apparatus was crude to the point of being ridiculous, Mosso's concept was sound and today is the basis of cutting-edge neuroimaging. FMRI measures the flow of blood to structures and areas within the brain when they're active, or functional.

Functional MRI is easy to fall in love with. I was enchanted with my first sight of an fMRI scan: a gray-scale picture of a cross section of a human brain, like a slice of the head taken parallel with the floor. The brain's anatomy was clearly visible in black and white, but patches in the occipital lobe at the back of the brain glowed brilliant yellow and orange to show activation of that area in response to a visual stimulus.

It was vertiginous, like looking in two mirrors reflecting each other: this picture allowed me to use my eyes to tell my brain what happens inside someone else's brain when they use their eyes to look at the world. I was only observing someone else's work, but it seemed like a miracle, a glimpse into the previously unknown. I felt the way Galileo must have when he looked through his telescope, or Armstrong when his foot hit the moon.

FMRI may be easy to love, but not to explain. When I asked Gabrieli how it works, he declined to answer, claiming a lack of expertise in the physics involved. Instead, he sent me to see his longtime collaborator, Dr. Gary Glover. Glover is a physicist and, before coming to Stanford, was a member of the team at General Electric that developed magnetic resonance imaging in the seventies. "You'll like him," Gabrieli told me. "He'll be wearing shorts."

Glover did greet me at the door of the seventeen-thousand-square-foot Lucas Center, Stanford's state-of-the-art MRI facility, of which he is the director, wearing khaki shorts and Birkenstock sandals. Right away he took me down to the basement of the center to see an fMRI scanner, which looked like a six-foot sugar cube with a hole bored through the center at waist height. The white cube is a refrigerator, which keeps the magnet inside it from overheating. That magnet is a metal coil, like a gigantic electrified—and thus magnetized—Slinky. The refrigerator and the coil surround a narrow platform that slides in and out of the hole in the center of the cube. A subject lies on the platform, with her head on a pillow made of Styrofoam beads. Once the subject's head is in place, a vacuum pump sucks all the air out from between the beads, making a rigid mold of the head and holding it completely still, as subjects must be absolutely motionless within the coffinlike center of the device, often for over an hour at a time, repeatedly performing mental tasks while their brains are scanned. That fact and the earsplitting racket the scanner makes as it works mean subjects must be carefully screened for claustrophobia.

While I was there, one of Gabrieli's students was working at a flat-panel monitor in the control room, separated from the scanner by a solid wall of glass. She was programming a series of pictures for that day's experiment; later those pictures would appear simultaneously on her display and on a similar display suspended within the scanner above the subject's head.

After the tour, Glover led me to his office and headed immediately for a whiteboard, covered from top to bottom with equations scribbled in red marker. He took an eraser, rubbed out a pie-size clearing in the middle of the board, and stood there, marker poised. "The basic idea," he told me, "is that people are weakly magnetic." And then the marker hit the board and he was off into spin.

It isn't possible to explain magnetic resonance imaging without first talking about an atomic quality physicists call spin, a feature of an atom's nucleus imparted to it by the electrons orbiting around it. For this reason it's hard to describe, as those electrons have both particle-like and wavelike properties. But it's easiest to get your mind around the concept if you imagine each atom as a spinning top. There is an axis around which the top spins, and that axis points in a particular direction. Not all atoms have nuclear spin—helium, for instance, as one of the noble gases, does not—but those that do have spin act as minuscule magnets in essentially the same way an electromagnet does: spinning electrical charges create a magnetic field that lies along the axis around which the charges spin.

Normally, the tiny spins of the atoms in your body have no net effect—your watch still works, compasses don't go haywire when you walk by—because the spin axes are all lying around randomly and so tend to cancel one another out. But if a person is placed in a strong magnetic field such as the one created by the coil of a magnetic resonance scanner, some of the spins move into alignment with that larger magnetic field, whose axis runs along the length of the platform on which the subject lies.

There are two ways in which an atom can align with the magnetic field: either parallel or antiparallel to it. The antiparallel configuration is slightly higher energy, meaning that it's more likely to change position; the difference between the two alignments is something like the difference between a quarter resting on its edge and one resting flat. A few atoms, just a couple per million, line up with their spins antiparallel to the magnetic field created by the scanner.

Once the atoms are lined up, either parallel or antiparallel to the larger magnetic field, you "perturb the system," as Glover put it, by hitting it with a radio-frequency pulse, a brief burst of a rotating magnetic field. The pulse provides enough energy to flip a few more of the atoms from the parallel toward the higher-energy antiparallel alignment. When the pulse ends, these flipped atoms relax back into the lower-energy state. The effect is as if many small magnets were tracing a path from one alignment to the other. MRI works by placing a sensor beside that path, so that it picks up the magnetic signal from the flipped atoms as they relax back down to the lower-energy state.

The scanner is set to detect one specific atom—usually hydrogen, as there's a lot of it in the human body in the form of water—and uses additional magnetic fields to tag the specific location of each hydrogen atom as it traces its path from the high- to the low-energy alignment. The scanner can then create an image based on the locations of those hydrogen atoms and the fact that they behave differently depending on the kind of tissue they're in—fat, bone, or muscle, for example.

With all this talk of atoms and alignments, it's easy to get lost in the theory and forget that what you're dealing with in an MRI scanner is a magnet with the same properties as the little doodads we stick on our refrigerators—albeit three hundred times stronger. Anyone who works with MRI quickly learns to leave her wallet outside the scanning room to avoid losing the information encoded in the magnetic strips of her credit cards. Neither researchers nor subjects can wear jewelry or metal hair clips, as they may be sucked right up into the magnet or simply get so hot from all the moving atoms that they burn their wearer. And the reason the Lucas Center had only flat-panel monitors long before they were widely used was not cosmetic. Traditional cathode-ray-tube screens "go all wonky," says Glover, because of the strong magnetic field.

Some people in particular shouldn't be exposed to the magnet. Glover gave the example of a patient who had worked in a machine shop prior to being scanned. It is not uncommon, he told me, for people who've worked in machine shops to have metal fragments lodged in their eyes, even without their knowing it. In this case, when the patient was put in the scanner and the magnet turned on, a splinter of metal he didn't know was in his eye moved into alignment with the scanner's magnetic field, nicking a blood vessel in the back of his eye on its way. No one knew this had happened, and the buildup of blood eventually compressed the retinal cells as they entered the optic nerve, resulting in blindness in that eye. "So," Glover told me, "every screening from then on has that kind of question in it: 'Have you ever worked in a machine shop?'"

Glover's explanation so far only brings us to magnetic resonance imaging, the sort of garden-variety MRI Roberta Glick uses in her practice to diagnose and monitor brain tumors. But for Glover and the "psychos"—as he calls Gabrieli and those more interested in the brain than in the science that allows them to look at it—the real fascination is with functional MRI. In fMRI, the basic image is created through MRI, and then thought processes are tracked via changes in that image caused by fluctuations in blood flow, with increased blood flow to a particular area of the brain reflecting increased activity in that spot.

In earlier functional brain-imaging techniques, such as positron-emission tomography (PET) scans, and even early fMRI, a patient or subject was injected with a contrast agent—a substance that would give off a traceable signal as it traveled around the body in the blood. But those agents are, for the most part, radioactive, meaning an increased risk of cancer with each injection. Repeat studies were virtually impossible, and studies in children rarely done. In the early 1990s, however, scientists at AT&T's Bell Laboratories came up with a way to measure blood flow based on properties of the blood itself. Hemoglobin, the molecule in the blood that carries oxygen, has significant magnetization only when it is not carrying oxygen. Deoxygenated blood is therefore highly magnetized and so interferes with the magnetic signal from the hydrogen in surrounding tissue, paradoxically causing a *reduction* in magnetic signal. Conversely, an influx of fresh, oxygenated (and thus less magnetized) blood to an area of the brain interferes less and *raises* the magnetic signal detectable from hydrogen in the surrounding tissue.

In other words, when Gabrieli's students put a subject in the scanner and show her pictures to learn what happens in her brain when she recognizes an image, the scanner records an increase in magnetic signal from the brain areas doing the recognizing. It is this difference in signal dependent on blood-oxygen level (the technique is called BOLD, for blood-oxygen-level dependent) that allows scientists to explore how and where we think.

Cognitive neuroscience is, as Glover said once he'd finished his explanation, "a big field," and since its development, fMRI—which because it is apparently harmless allows for study of children's brains and repeated adult experiments—has been used to study questions as varied as where in our brains we experience emotion, how arachnophobes' brains react to spiders, and how damaged brains like the baby's on which Glick operated reorganize to function normally. The tools Glover uses to aid scholars in that big field are also big: As he walked me out of the Lucas Center, which he helped design, Glover said, "See that hatch?" pointing through a wall of glass to a ten-foot-square steel lid set in the ground. He told me parts of the center's fMRI scanner had been lowered by crane through the hatch to reach its basement resting place. One of those parts was the magnet itself, which, he said, weighs about thirteen and a half tons.

GLOVER AND HIS enormous magnet arrived at Stanford at almost the same time Gabrieli's circuitous career path landed him there. Although he was an English literature major at Yale in the 1970s, Gabrieli told me he had nevertheless planned to be a doctor like his father, who was a surgeon and clinical pathologist. "As long as I can remember, that was the thing I planned on being," he told me. "I think because my father was a physician and that was well spoken of."

It certainly must have been. Sometime during the days I spent with Gabrieli, I spoke with his mother on the phone from Boston. She couldn't say enough about doctors and doctoring. Upon learning that I was in medical school, she said, "Oh, there is nothing more beautiful, believe me, nothing. We thought John would be a doctor, but he was so decided to go into research. We weren't delighted with it, believe me. It was very unexpected. But he just got carried away."

What carried Gabrieli away was the study of human memory. After graduating from Yale, he got a job in Dr. Suzanne Corkin's lab at MIT. Around the time Gabrieli joined her, Corkin was performing a series of groundbreaking experiments on memory that followed in the footsteps of the pioneering Canadian scientist Dr. Brenda

Milner. Many of those experiments focused on one person, a man Gabrieli refers to as "the noted patient HM."

HM is famous among those who study the brain and the mind, although he himself doesn't know it. As a teenager and well into his twenties, HM suffered from debilitating epilepsy, experiencing dozens of seizures a day. In 1953, when he was twenty-seven, HM decided to undergo surgery to remove the area of his brain where the seizures began. For the operation, he was referred to Dr. William Scoville, a man alternately lauded and reviled in the mountains of literature about HM's case but who, through his treatment of HM and subsequent decision to make public the grievous results of that treatment, has probably contributed more to the understanding of memory than any other scholar.

When Scoville prepared to operate on HM, he was, in a sense, flying in the dark. Surgery for epilepsy was not new: the first such operation (which was successful) had been performed almost seventy years earlier. But Scoville had been unable to localize where in HM's brain the seizures started, so he didn't really know which part of the brain he ought to remove. A common place for seizures to begin in epileptics, however, is the hippocampus, an area within the temporal lobe:

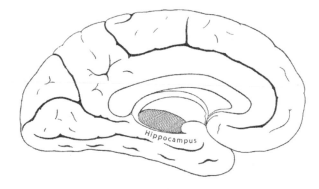

This is a sagittal section, a slice taken parallel to a line drawn
from the nose to the back of the head along the midline.

The hippocampus, like almost all structures in the brain, is really two structures, one in each hemisphere. In the absence of other information, Scoville chose to remove HM's hippocampus, considering it the most likely focus of his seizures. Because he didn't even know on which side of HM's brain the seizures were beginning, Scoville chose to remove the hippocampus bilaterally. He also took out portions of the brain near the hippocampus on both sides; the entire area from which Scoville removed tissue is known collectively as the medial temporal lobe and comprises the hippocampus and structures known as the amygdala and the uncus.

HM is still alive today, and in a sense Scoville's operation was a success: HM's epilepsy, most agree, is better. But as Gabrieli says, there was "this tremendous side effect" of the surgery, "which has gotten him into every psychology textbook and medical textbook that's published, which is: For all practical purposes, from that day forward to the present, he has not been able to remember a new event or a new fact for more than a few seconds."

HM can no longer make any new conscious memories. Because of his case and research sparked by it, we now know that the hippocampus is vital to our capacity to create and store memories, although science is just beginning to study how exactly it performs those functions.

At the same time that HM's horrible outcome made clear the importance of the hippocampus to memory, it also made it clear that the hippocampus isn't the only part of the brain that allows us to remember who we are and what has happened to us. HM can easily tell you stories from his childhood, can tell you who the president was when he started high school, can recognize celebrities famous when he was growing up and sing songs from that time — in short, he has a full set of memories of his life until a few years before his surgery.

That he is missing memories even from years before the surgery gives credence to one theory of the hippocampus's role in memory consolidation, which is that the record your brain keeps of experiences stays in the hippocampus for years before being transferred—maybe gradually, maybe all at once—to other parts of the brain. Terry Dibert's case also supports that theory. After the police identified him, Dibert was taken to a hospital in Pennsylvania, where he was diagnosed with a benign fluid-filled cyst that had been pressing on a part of his brain called the fornix. The fornix serves as a pathway from the hippocampus to other parts of the brain, and it may be that the cyst blocked the flow of information along it. Such a blockage would prevent Dibert from accessing more recent memories stored in the hippocampus, yet would still allow him to retrieve older memories consolidated and stored elsewhere.

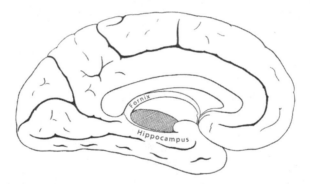

Once the cyst was drained, most of Dibert's newer memories returned, but HM was not so lucky. He is now in his seventies, yet he cannot remember where he has lived during the last sixty years or so. He cannot remember anyone he has met since years before his surgery, or even what he had for lunch half an hour ago. "He doesn't know that men have gone to the moon," Gabrieli says. "His parents have passed away, and he doesn't know. No matter how dramatic an event's personal consequences, no matter how publicly discussed, they are all a blank to him."*

---

* HM's particular brand of amnesia has inspired any number of books and movies, some of them more scientifically accurate than others. In *50 First Dates*, for

What he can do is talk, push buttons, and report his sensations and memories—or lack thereof—as any human can and no mouse or monkey, no matter how well trained, is able to. Thus HM, a quiet Catholic boy from Connecticut with an eighth-grade education, revolutionized the study of memory. "Before HM," Gabrieli told me, "most research on amnesics was just documenting how really *bad* their memory was. For years and years that was it." But now science had a patient with an unusually "pure" amnesia—HM showed no signs of dementia or other brain damage—and what's more, the exact location of his brain lesion was known. And "he's an excellent subject for experiments," Gabrieli says. "Most subjects we run, three minutes into the experiment they're checking their watch—the fun's over, now come trials three through nine thousand. But he's awesome because he has no idea that he's been doing something for a while. Boredom is meaningless to him; he only knows the last five seconds of his life." Which means that researchers—who sometimes seem to share this boredom deficit—are able to sit with HM for hours, showing him pictures, numbers, or words and testing his memory for those pictures, numbers, or words five seconds, ten seconds, thirty seconds, minutes, hours, days, or years later.

It may seem inhumane to use HM in this way. It's a conundrum: His intelligence is completely intact, so he can understand and sign an informed consent, and he does for each experiment. But he has no way of knowing that it's the twentieth, thirtieth, or hundredth such form he's been presented with. However, besides the fact that there

---

example, the conceit is that Drew Barrymore's character has a similar amnesia following brain damage incurred during a car accident. Conveniently for the plot, she is able to retain memories over the course of a day, allowing her to have some kind of meaningful relationship with her swain, played by Adam Sandler. In reality, of course, even in the unlikely event that a car accident had caused bilateral medial temporal lobe damage, her disability would be more like that of HM and of Ten Second Tom, another character in the movie. Ten Second Tom is played only for laughs and can't carry on even a simple conversation because by the time he's finished introducing himself, he's already forgotten that he's done so.

is a clear and enormous benefit to science gained by studying HM, Gabrieli points out that it's senseless to think of him as you would another, normal subject. "You could be mean, if you wanted, and explain to him, 'Your memory is like the worst anybody's had. You're in all the textbooks as a horrible memory person,' right? But by the time you're on your third or fourth sentence, he's already fading on the first sentence, and moments later he won't remember it anyway."

Because Gabrieli worked directly with HM, his lectures are often reduced for long stretches to impromptu discussions of HM's predicament. He never seems to tire of the topic, however, answering all questions with the same sense of raw wonder in which they are invariably posed. At one lecture I attended, during which easily twenty minutes were spent with hands waving in the air, Gabrieli fielded a query about HM's feelings on his own appearance, given that he can't remember all the years he's lived to bring him to his current age. "Excellent question," Gabrieli said. "Does he look into the mirror every day and shriek?" It turns out he doesn't: somehow, despite the fact that when asked, HM will guess his age to be somewhere in his twenties or early thirties, some part of his brain has gotten used to the face of an old man gazing out from his reflection. Asked about HM's personal growth, Gabrieli said, "As far as one can tell, he's had no change in personality or emotional growth or anything. Now"— with a smile—"many people are identified as being childish in their forties, fifties, and seventies, so it's hard to actually prove that."*

In that lecture, Gabrieli used HM to illustrate the theory of multiple memory systems, as his case provided some of the basis for the model. The significance of the experiments that did so was not immediately recognized, however. In the early 1960s, long before Gabrieli was to work with her, Brenda Milner put HM through a

---

* Gabrieli is known for his dry sense of humor. At a conference I attended, one speaker introduced her talk by describing how she'd run into him the day before and had mentioned the subject of her talk, which was Alzheimer's disease. "Are you going to be very controversial," he asked her, "and come out against it?"

standard battery of tests of brain and memory function and noticed that on certain kinds of tasks he didn't do any worse than people with normal memories. One of those tasks was mirror drawing: subjects were taught to trace between two lines on a piece of paper while watching their hands only in a mirror. A person with a normal brain will be terrible at mirror drawing initially, then gradually improve as her brain correlates messages from the eyes with the signals it must send the muscles in order to achieve the required hand movements. Normal subjects will also, of course, consciously remember having practiced the skill.

HM, on the other hand, does not remember ever having performed it before, though he's probably done it scores of times by now. Each time he has to have the rules explained to him all over again. But in what must have been one of the eerier moments in science, Milner and her team noticed that HM nonetheless got better at staying within the lines. He got better at the same rate, in fact, as normal subjects.

When Milner's results were published, the neuroscience community's reaction to this news about HM was equivocal. Not much was concluded about memory as a whole. It wasn't until 1980—when, among other developments, Dr. Neal Cohen and Dr. Larry Squire, at the University of California at San Diego, published a paper with the precise if unwieldy title "Preserved Learning and Retention of Pattern-Analyzing Skill in Amnesia: Dissociation of Knowing How and Knowing That" in the journal *Science*—that there was a paradigm shift in how scientists think about human memory. Cohen and Squire stated clearly and courageously their belief, based on Milner's data and their own experiments showing normal improvement in reading of mirror-image words by people with amnesia, that "amnesia seems to spare information that is based on rules or procedures, as contrasted with information that is data-based or declarative."

In other words, they believed there to be at least two memory systems, of which our conscious memory—the memory we use to recall past experiences, traditionally considered the whole of memory—is only one. Squire wrote years later that "this finding broadened the scope of what amnesic patients could do, and suggested a major distinction between declarative forms of memory, which are impaired in amnesia, and non-declarative forms of memory, which are preserved in amnesia."

And that, to this day, is the basic distinction between what scientists refer to as declarative memory and nondeclarative memory: If amnesics can do it, it relies on nondeclarative memory systems. If they can't, it's a function of declarative processes. Gabrieli admits that such a definition is problematic. No one knows where in the brain nondeclarative memories are produced or stored, and there's no independent definition of either declarative or nondeclarative memory, although in general, declarative memory is defined as conscious recollections of events or information, and nondeclarative memory refers to physical or cognitive skills. What definitions do exist are still under debate, in a field so riddled with overlapping terminology that Endel Tulving, a kind of patriarch of modern memory research, once wrote a paper in which he felt it necessary to include a table correlating the terms used by different investigators for different types of memory (for example, declarative memory is sometimes called episodic, semantic, or explicit, and nondeclarative memory is also known as procedural or implicit).

One of the nondeclarative forms of memory Gabrieli studied in HM and in normal control subjects, and continues to study today with the help of fMRI, is a phenomenon called priming. To understand priming, imagine taking two groups of subjects and showing a list of words to group A. The list might include, among others, the words *stamp, landmark, speak,* and *clock.* Group B doesn't get a list. Later, you give everyone in both groups a list of word stems, like this: *sta——, tem——, lan——, sen——,* and ask them to complete the stems with any word they'd like, telling group A that the stems have no relation to the list they were previously given. However, most of the subjects in group A, having seen the list, will add *mp* to the first stem to make *stamp,* and the third they'll complete as *landmark.* There will be normal variation in responses completing the other stems. The subjects in group B, who didn't see a previous word list, will also have normal variation in completing the *sta* and *lan* stems.

This finding demonstrates that recent sight of the words *land-mark* and *stamp* had somehow made those words more accessible in the minds of those in group A. That discovery isn't remarkable in normal subjects, as you might assume they're consciously remembering having seen those words recently. But as Gabrieli says, "You'll tell HM that the word stems have no relation to the first word list, and he'll say, 'What first list?'" Yet HM and other amnesics will still tend to fill in the previously seen words when presented with the appropriate stems, despite having no conscious recollection of seeing the words. This phenomenon, which can be demonstrated in other ways, is known as priming and refers to, as Gabrieli has written, "a change in the processing of a stimulus, usually words or pictures, due to prior exposure to the same or related stimulus."

Priming and amnesics' ability to acquire skills without consciously remembering their acquisition were discovered before the development of fMRI, but since then Gabrieli and others have tried to use the technology to learn where such memories are stored. While such work is still under way, both priming and improvement at skilled tasks appear to be accompanied by activation changes in brain areas related to the sense used in the study task. For instance, Gabrieli's group did an fMRI experiment with auditory priming in which they asked subjects to determine whether a recorded sound (of a dog barking or a door slamming, for example) had been made by an animal or not. Subjects demonstrated priming by responding more quickly to sounds they had heard before than to sounds they hadn't. In those cases, their auditory cortices showed a *decrease* in activation, a finding that has been interpreted to mean that the repetition of the sound had somehow made the auditory cortex more efficient at processing it, even when the subject herself was unaware of having previously heard the sound.

There are other instances in which our brains appear to be processing stimuli without our awareness. Gabrieli's research has expanded beyond memory in part because he makes it a policy to let his students explore areas they find interesting. It was one such student who convinced Gabrieli to let him use fMRI to explore olfaction and who then demonstrated that inhaled chemicals can affect the brain without consciously being smelled. In those experiments, a compound called oestra-1,3,5(10),16-tetraen-3yl acetate was spritzed into a "sniff halter," a contraption that fit over subjects' noses and allowed them to inhale the pure compound. The subjects claimed to detect no odor whatsoever. Yet on fMRI, their brains showed significant activation in certain precise areas — the same areas in all subjects tested — when the substance was introduced. How does this happen? What allows a compound to be consciously recognized as a smell? What effect do the unconsciously neuroactive substances have? It is this kind of mystery that Gabrieli loves and that fMRI helps him to unlock.

The discovery of priming, the work showing that amnesics have intact skill learning, and subsequent research hinting at even more types of unconscious learning and detection are leading to a new understanding of both memory and consciousness, one Gabrieli compares to a symphony orchestra. "All of the brain is a learning machine," he says, "but each part is learning in its own way and for its own domain of knowledge." What those ways are and where that learning happens are still under investigation. Nevertheless, such findings have made a big splash among those interested in the mind, since some interpret them to be scientific evidence for Freud's cognitive unconscious. Although it is generally spurned by modern scientists as superstition, there are those who believe Freud's theory is showing new merit in light of these developments. It now appears, Gabrieli said, that just as Freud thought, "we might be moving around daily, driven by these kinds of memories all the time, but we don't even realize it's a memory that's driving us to do something or believe something or say something." It's possible, he suggests, that "we're operating on a system that doesn't even know where we learned something, just like HM."

Conception	6 weeks	10 weeks	30 weeks	6 years	Adolescence	Adulthood	Old Age	Death

Birth

S ometime after beginning their trip from the inner surface of your neural tube to the outer surface of what would become your brain, your neurons—which until then had been simple sacks of cytoplasm— began to sprout little processes:

In each neuron, one of these processes began to grow faster than the others, becoming the long, thin axon, the main route along which a neuron sends out messages. The rest of the processes became the neurons' dendrites, which receive messages from other neurons. Roughly speaking, if a neuron were a radio, the axon would be the speakers and the dendrites the receiver.

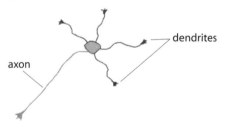

dendrites

axon

As they grew, your neurons' axons began to seek out the other neurons with which they would connect to form synapses. Those target neurons might be far away: there are axons that run the length of the brain, and axons that travel from the brain far down into the spinal cord. A neuron in your visual cortex, located in the occipital lobe at the back of your head, might have to send its axon many centimeters forward to the fusiform gyrus, where visual information will be needed for face recognition.

In order to find its target, an axon has to bob and weave among all the other neurons in its path, as if it were a concertgoer hunting for a friend in a packed crowd. Like a newly arrived rock fan in search of her buddies, the axon sets out apparently at random, its only imperative to keep moving. Supporting it in its mission is the neuron cell body, which assembles and packages food and building materials and sends them forward along the axon, allowing it to grow as it seeks its target.

Although it begins creeping forward blindly, the tip of an axon may soon encounter molecules called semaphorins. Semaphorins nearly always act as repellents, sending the axon off in a different direction. In a developing brain, some semaphorins are made by cells at the outer edge of the brain and send growing axons deep into the brain. So semaphorins, like impatient concertgoers at the back of the crowd, tend to push the axon along its path.

En route, axons also encounter "guideposts." Acting like mutual acquaintances in the mob at a concert ("Gwen? Yeah, I saw her. She was headed that way"), these guidepost cells make semaphorins or other signal molecules that direct the axon tip to change direction. Located every few micrometers, the guideposts effectively break the long voyage of the axon into hundreds or thousands of tiny steps.

After one axon has taken a particular route through the growing brain, axons from other neurons—like friends following a leader through a throng of music fans—will tend to latch onto the trailblazer axon and follow the already-beaten path.

On reaching their target areas around the brain, many axons split into branches. Those branches seek the dendrites of other nearby neurons to synapse on.* Once they find another neuron's dendrites, multiple vesicles collect at the ends of the axons' branches. Those vesicles are something like the little condom balls filled with cocaine that drug mules

---

* This is something of an oversimplification. An axonal branch can actually synapse anywhere on another neuron — its cell body, its dendrites, even along the length of its axon. But for the most part, dendrites are post-synaptic areas and receive information, and axons are presynaptic terminals and release information.

swallow, with a layer of cell membrane in place of the latex, and a neuro-transmitter in place of the cocaine.

The vesicles sit inside the neuron, tethered in grapelike clusters to the cell membrane at the end of the axon. With the right signal, one or a few of the vesicles are released, allowing the vesicles' membranes to fuse with the cell membrane of the neuron in which they're contained. That fusing spills the molecules of neurotransmitter from the vesicle out of the cell altogether. Those molecules float out into the synaptic cleft—the space between the axon releasing the neurotransmitter and the den-drites picking it up. The dendrites on the receiving or postsynaptic neuron have receptors for the neurotransmitter; a molecule of neurotransmitter bumping into one of those receptors will bind to it, causing a change in the postsynaptic neuron.

It is in this way that your neurons found one another and began to communicate. Despite the painstaking process by which each axon was forced to find its synaptic target, such connections were made at a stag-gering rate. When you were a seven-and-a-half-month-old fetus, about forty thousand synapses were created in your brain each second.

I just think that consciousness, as we can understand it, is brain function.

—JOHN GABRIELI

3 | Mining the Brain

"FRANCIS, HAVE I SHOWED you this amazing movie?" asked Dr. Christof Koch. He is tall, lanky, and, because of his passion for rock climbing, muscular for a man of his age (forty-eight) and occupation (neuroscientist). While Koch's hair is naturally brown peppered with gray, it was dyed pomegranate red that day. He and I were sitting in the kitchen at the La Jolla home of his collaborator, Francis Crick, who long before teaming up with Koch worked with James Watson to discover the helical structure of DNA. We—Koch, Crick, Crick's wife, Odile, and I—had just finished a lunch of poached salmon, salad, and apple tart but were still gathered around the table. "I'm going to put it on my Web site," Koch said, turning around his laptop* so Crick could see the movie, "with a U2 song to go with it."

The son of diplomats, Koch grew up in Germany, Holland,

---

* Koch's laptop is a Macintosh PowerBook. "If any OS becomes conscious, it'll be a Mac," he said to me once. He has also written that "together with the Boeing B-747 Jumbo Jet and the Golden Gate Bridge in San Francisco, the Apple Macintosh is the most beautiful and elegant artifact of the 20th century. A perfect marriage of form with function." His devotion to the Mac is so great that he has a tattoo of the multicolored Apple logo on his right shoulder.

Canada, and Morocco and didn't learn English until he was a teenager in Ottawa, although he was born in Kansas City, Missouri ("Cahn't you heeah the ahccent?" he asks). In addition to his German accent, Koch leaves out articles when he's excited, which is nearly all the time. "Isn't this amazing movie?" he asked.

Crick leaned forward across the table, his eyes intent under bushy white brows. He was eighty-seven and already quite ill with the cancer that killed him ten months later. "Hey, that's very interesting," he said, peering at Koch's computer.

The movie was only a few seconds long. It showed a gray and black image of a heart, the walls rhythmically contracting. The heart belonged, it turned out, to Koch, and the image was captured by a new functional MRI technique. "It goes through two heartbeats, and it's amazing how accurate it is," Koch said. "It's a huge organ—I hadn't realized it—the heart. It's fifteen centimeters."*

"Hmmm," Crick said. He then turned to me and, in the English accent startling to those of us whose mental image of him was created by reading *The Double Helix,* written by the Chicago-born James Watson with a certain American flair, said, "I don't suppose you've noticed the influence of Aristotle on everyday life?"

His question made me nervous. A fierce intellect and a vigorous upholder of the scientific method, Crick didn't suffer fools gladly, and before we met, Koch had written to warn me that Crick only agreed to interviews "provided that the author/journalist has sufficient background on the subject at hand (i.e., he doesn't like to be interviewed by English majors that don't know the difference between DNA and RNA) and that what they write (or have written in the past) is serious, science-based (as compared to being very fluffy)."

Three hours into our afternoon together, DNA and RNA hadn't

---

* The image can be seen by following a link in the Web content area of www .shannonmoffett.com.

been a problem. But already I had irritated Crick by asking him about solipsism (the idea that everything in the world is a figment of one's imagination), which he considered foolishness; I had gotten him riled up about the philosopher Daniel Dennett's work, featured in chapter 6, which he considered lacking in scientific rigor; and I had found myself telling him about an article mentioning his name that I'd found on the *Washington Post*'s Web site. The ensuing exchange—with Francis Crick, a Nobel Prize–winning scientist and father of molecular biology—went like this:

> ME: So I clicked on the link, and it said, "Brownies, Cakey or Fudgy?"
> CRICK: What?!
> ME: Brownies—you know, the little treats?
> CRICK (*with a dangerous look in his eye*): Yes?
> ME: Um, so I read this whole thing about whether the feature writer, you know, prefers cakey or fudgy brownies. And at the bottom she's talking about a cookbook written by a woman who she says "has decided to do for chocolate what Jim Watson and Francis Crick did for DNA."*

Luckily for me, both Koch and Odile burst into peals of laughter, and even Crick chuckled. Now, though, worried I've used up his forbearance, and knowing I can't produce a single quote from Aristotle and that if I could I would have no idea how it influences us in daily life, I just looked at him.

"Because," he said, "you see these signs that say I—and then

---

* The real headline for Candy Sagon's article in the *Washington Post*'s food section, October 8, 2003, was CAKEY VS. FUDGY. And her line about the chocolate maven Alice Medrich, far better than my rendition of it, was "she has applied herself to cracking the mysteries of chocolate the way James Watson and Francis Crick took on DNA."

there's a heart—LA JOLLA. I love La Jolla. But that was Aristotle that thought the brain was in the heart, you see. Well, he got it wrong."

Aristotle, of course, thought the *mind* was in the heart, but for Crick the words *mind* and *brain* were synonymous, although he always admitted that posited synonymity remains unproven. In 1994, he published a book titled *The Astonishing Hypothesis*. Its first sentence is "The Astonishing Hypothesis is that 'You,' your joys and your sorrows, your memories and your ambitions, your sense of personal identity and free will, are in fact no more than the behavior of a vast assembly of nerve cells and their associated molecules." Crick goes on to say we ought to study the brain not only to cure illness but "to grasp the true nature of the human soul," adding that "whether this term is metaphorical or literal is exactly what we are trying to discover." Thus the book's subtitle, *The Scientific Search for the Soul.* It was in that search that Crick and Koch were engaged.

But what was the genteel but hard-nosed English physicist who helped describe the elegantly paired and winding DNA molecule doing in Southern California, studying the traditionally fuzzy and scientifically eschewed subject of consciousness? The answer, as Crick had told me earlier in the day, goes back a long way.

WHEN I'D ARRIVED that morning, Koch had appeared moments after Odile let me into the kitchen of the Cricks' long white stucco ranch. He walked me the length of the house, past windows looking out onto a leafy yard and swimming pool, to Crick's study. Crick was waiting for us there, dressed in tan trousers, a button-down shirt and a burgundy sweater, his commanding height concealed by the fact that he was sitting far back on a low sofa, a walking stick by his knee. He gave me a firm handshake while Koch seated himself in a chair in the corner opposite him.

"As far back as I can remember," he told me once we were settled, "I always wanted to be a scientist." The kind of kid who apparently read cover-to-cover the children's encyclopedia given him by his parents—whom he later dismayed by using his chemistry set to blow up bottles in the family's basement. Crick eventually settled on physics as his branch of science. He graduated from University College in London with a physics degree and entered graduate school at twenty-one years old, working on "this very dull problem given to me by a professor—how to measure the viscosity of water at temperatures above a hundred degrees centigrade."

The problem involved constructing a spherical copper vessel to hold the water. It had to be built to exact specifications, perfectly round, with a neck to allow the water to expand when heated, at which point, using films of the water's decaying oscillations as it cooled, its viscosity could be calculated. "I mean, I ask you," Crick said to me, rolling his eyes.

So he was relieved when, after World War II broke out, his entire department relocated to Wales. He stayed behind in London, where he worked for the Admiralty, roughly the equivalent of the navy in the United States. Although he worked in a couple of different departments there, including scientific intelligence ("to discover what the Russians were doing in science"), Crick spent much of the time in the Mine Design Department, working on making underwater acoustic and magnetic mines capable of going undiscovered by enemy minesweepers. How fitting, then, that when the war ended, he learned his copper vessel had been destroyed by a land mine.

Although he was by then almost thirty, Crick was able to see both the loss of his ill-fated bottle and his lack of experience—he had published no scientific papers—as opportunities, and he set about finding a more interesting path. After several months of "brooding" over what to do next, he realized that two topics kept cropping up in his idle conversations with friends. One was where exactly the border between living and nonliving things could be found, a topic of great interest at the time. The other subject he found himself returning to again and again was the puzzle of how the human brain works. "In both cases," Crick told me, "I thought there was a deep mystery there which hadn't been solved."

Lucky enough to realize he should pick one of these two areas to work in, given that they fascinated him enough to qualify as café-chat material, he reasoned that his background in physics (not to mention his habit of covertly reading an organic chemistry textbook behind his desk at the Admiralty) made him more qualified for what he at the time called the "chemical physics of biology" (what we would today call molecular biology) than for studying the brain.

Having made the decision, Crick was immediately tempted to re-think it when he was offered a job in a lab studying vision. The scien-tist who made the offer was working to prove his hypothesis that the human eye has as many as seven different types of cones, the color-sensing cells in the retina. (That turned out to be false: most people have only three kinds, although about 7 percent of men have only two cone types and many women have four types.) As Crick later wrote in *What Mad Pursuit,* a memoir of his life in science, the scientist also "seemed to me a little too bouncy, and I was not completely sure we would get on."

He refused the job, deciding to hold out for another ("I had no idea it would work out so well," he says now, mildly), and was even-tually offered one, in a lab at the University of Cambridge. There he spent a year or two studying chick fibroblasts, a kind of cell that could be induced to engulf and take up a tiny piece of metal. The bit of metal would then move around inside the cell when it was put under a magnetic field, allowing Crick to deduce information about the properties of the cell's cytoplasm, the fluid inside the cell.

While the job sounds hardly more interesting than the water-viscosity problem, Crick said the work was easy enough that he was able to educate himself about genetics and organic molecules at the same time, so that in 1951 when a chance came to move to the Physics

Department at Cambridge—known as the Cavendish Laboratory—
to study proteins using X-ray diffraction, he was ready, if not formally
qualified. "Imagine," he says now, "getting into the leading physics lab
in the country without any publications."

What Crick brought instead of publications was a wide-ranging
intelligence that seems to have impressed all who met him. Robert
Olby, who is working on a biography of Crick, has studied papers and
correspondence from Crick's past, including his file at England's
Medical Research Council, under whose auspices Crick did his work
at Cambridge. The file includes documents from as far back as when
he was interviewing for positions. "His story," said Crick of Olby, "is
that he actually found their comments on me at the time."

And?

"They said sort of, well, 'He seems bright, we like him.'"

"They said 'promising,' in one case," Koch chimed in.

Which Olby confirmed when I sent him an e-mail, adding that
all who interviewed Crick were clearly taken with him. "This is evident not only in what they wrote but in the prompt manner in which
they dealt with his application for support," Olby wrote.

The true promise Crick held couldn't have been evident at the
time, however, and in fact it got him in trouble. Still a graduate student at thirty-six, Crick was at the Cavendish Lab when he met Dr.
James Watson, who arrived there not long after he did. Twelve years
Crick's junior, Watson had nevertheless finished his PhD in zoology
two years earlier. Despite the disparity in their ages and academic ac-
complishments, the two clicked. They also found they agreed that
genes might well be contained in deoxyribonucleic acid, something
not universally accepted at the time.

That speculation was almost utterly irrelevant to what either one
was supposed to be doing while at the Cavendish. Crick's task was to
use X-ray diffraction to study the structure of proteins, not DNA.
Watson had come to Cambridge to work on crystallizing myoglobin,

a protein found in muscle, so that it could by studied by Crick. Their shared conviction concerning DNA had about as much to do with these two tasks as a shared love of crossword puzzles would have, but they began working together in their free time to find the structure of deoxyribonucleic acid—studying chemistry, building models, and, ironically enough, not actually doing any X-ray diffraction of DNA themselves. In fact, Crick was neglecting his diffraction duties, and says he was told at least once to quit messing around with Watson and get back to his official task of making pictures of proteins.

The command slowed the two down, but they kept at their extracurricular project whenever they could. Watson was eventually shown an X-ray diffraction image of DNA made by Rosalind Franklin, who was working with Maurice Wilkins, whom Crick had met during the job hunt that landed him at the chick cytoplasm lab. It was Franklin's picture that helped the pieces Crick and Watson had gathered during their illicit quest fall into place, leading to the duo's two famous papers in the journal *Nature* detailing their proposed double-helical-structure for DNA. Their structure, of course, turned out to be the correct one and led to an explanation of how genetic information is passed down through generations and how life is built from the lifeless molecules of which we are made.

The discovery, made in 1953, launched Crick's career. He spent almost a quarter of a century after that studying what is now called molecular biology, along with its logical offshoot, developmental biology. But in 1976, when he moved from Cambridge to San Diego's Salk Institute and was in a position to do whatever he wanted, Crick chose to revisit the fork in the road he'd faced at the end of World War II. "I was sixty," he told me, "no, a bit later. Anyway, an 'it's now or never' sort of thing." He decided to study the brain and consciousness.

Not long after that, Crick went to Tübingen, Germany, to visit Dr. Tomaso Poggio, whose work had piqued his interest. Poggio was then a professor at the Max Planck Institute for Biological Cybernetics and was studying dendritic spines, little outpouchings on the dendrites of a neuron.

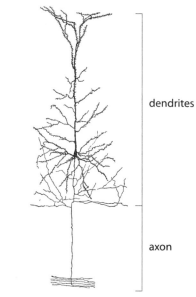

dendrites

axon

© *by Ramon y Cajal's heirs*

The dendritic spines, which Koch likes to compare to thorns on a rose,
can be seen here as tiny dots on the axon and dendrites.

Dendritic spines are still a mystery today. They seem to be the spots on the postsynaptic neuron that receive information from the presynaptic neuron, but they are so dynamic—changing shape and size and on occasion actually appearing and disappearing within the course of hours—that there is speculation (and some evidence) that they represent the brain's mechanism of learning.

When Crick arrived in Tübingen, Koch was in his twenties, sporting a couple of scars from the days when he engaged in Mensur Fechten, the traditional form of fencing duels using actual blades and little protective gear that was still practiced by university students in Germany when Koch was there. His new and safer passion was ballet, which to his regret he didn't discover until he was nineteen, too late to study it seriously. When not dancing, Koch was working on his PhD thesis on information processing in dendrites with Poggio as his advisor ("Doctor-father, as we say in Germany"). And so Crick and Koch met and struck up a friendship, which evolved into a collaboration after Koch finished his PhD and came to this country to begin work on visual processing in the brain.

Which is how, more than twenty-five years after turning his back on a job studying the visual system with a bouncy neuroscientist, Crick came to be studying the visual system with a crimson-haired, tattooed, rock-climbing maverick neuroscientist who could accurately be described as bouncy and with whom, despite that, Crick seems to get on famously.

MOST SCIENTISTS TODAY accept the hypothesis Crick dubbed astonishing: that consciousness arises solely from the activity of brain cells. When Crick and Koch began to work together, however, they took this hypothesis a step further. Given that a good deal of what happens in our brains is unavailable to our conscious minds — as work like the experiments done with HM has shown — Crick and Koch surmised that there must, somewhere in our brains, be certain mechanisms active when we are conscious and not active when we aren't. They thought it likely that those mechanisms arise from certain populations of neurons. But where are those cells? And how many of them are there? And what is it they *do* that is consciousness? No one knows, but the two were determined to find out. They called those cells and mechanisms the neural correlates of consciousness (thus allowing the possibility that the astonishing hypothesis is wrong by suggesting that those cells and mechanisms might simply be correlated with consciousness rather than the sole basis for it) and made searching for the NCC their mission.

Such a mission has not always been viewed kindly by the scientific community. At a meeting of the Association for the Scientific

Study of Consciousness that I attended, Dr. Bernard Baars, a cognitive neuroscientist and one of the organizers of the meeting, showed a graph he'd made based on a search of the scientific literature published since 1965. That year was what Baars calls "the height of behaviorism," when only measurable behavior was considered a fit subject for science, and scientists scoffed at anyone who talked about what might be going on in the minds of the animals they studied, even when those animals happened to be human. Baars searched the literature for the words *conscious, consciousness,* and a few similar terms. In 1965 there were almost no authors who dared to use any of the terms in his search. And between 1965 and 1970, the number of mentions of the subject of consciousness stayed about the same—essentially zero. But then, as the behaviorists lost ground, the number began to skyrocket, until in the year 2000 there were over five thousand articles that included one of the terms on Baars's list.

Even corrected for the increase since the mid-twentieth century in the overall number of scientific articles published on any subject, the rise in consciousness research has been meteoric. But in Crick and Koch's opinion, most of today's work on the subject has too broad a focus.

As we talked in Crick's office, Koch had begun thumbing through a book by the philosopher John Searle he'd pulled from the floor-to-ceiling bookcase behind him. Now he pointed from the top to the bottom of the bookcase. "All of these books, this entire shelf," he said, "from there to there, is all about consciousness. Every one of these books is on consciousness; you can see from the titles."

"And that's only a fraction of them," Crick said.

"OK, now, and the vast majority of these," Koch went on, "*Consciousness, The Neuroscience of Consciousness, Concept of the Mind, Beyond Dissociation*— the vast majority of these all deal at the philosophical or at the psychological level. Or some of the more recent ones, they'll talk a little bit about functional imaging or clinical data.

Which is great, but it's still at the very crude level—you're talking about this part of the brain versus that chunk of the brain versus that chunk of the brain."

Those chunks are called voxels. Matt Kirschen, a classmate of mine who works with fMRI, gave me a way to visualize them. "Take the entire brain," he said, "and divide it into one millimeter by one millimeter by one millimeter pieces so the entire brain looks like a giant Lego set, with one millimeter by one millimeter by one millimeter Legos. Each Lego is a voxel." The limit to how finely fMRI can discriminate between parts of the brain is dictated by the size of those voxels, and the smallest voxel manageable by today's fMRI scanners is about one cubic millimeter, and most fMRI work measures activity over multiple voxels. Koch later told me he'd once measured a grain of rice and found it to have a volume of eight cubic millimeters. In a piece of cortex that size, he said, there would be "close to a million neurons, and close to twenty kilometers—twelve miles of wires" if you laid each axon of those million neurons end-to-end. But they're not laid end-to-end, of course; they are interconnecting. And so, in that one grain of rice, if it were made of cortical brain tissue, you'd have, he said, "close to eight billion synapses."

As Koch pointed out, "Functional imaging is fantastic, and EEG and MEG,* it's all great, but we're looking at very, very bulk brain activity, right?" When using those techniques, he said, "it's a bit like you're up in space and you want to know what people are doing—you want to know what you and I are doing—to understand human society, but you can only track the power consumption on the electric grid. So what you see: In the evening, people go home, you know, turn on stoves, air-conditioning. Over the summer it gets hotter, air-conditioning goes

---

* EEG is electroencephalography, and MEG is magnetoencephalography. Both are noninvasive techniques that, like fMRI, record gross shifts in brain activity. EEG and MEG, however, measure neurons' electric action; fMRI measures blood flow. Thus fMRI has better spatial resolution, but EEG and MEG are faster.

up, things like that." You could get some useful information from such an anthropologic study, he said, but if you want to know something about the relationship between the sexes, for instance, or between employees and bosses, or teenagers and their parents, you need to look at activity on a smaller scale.

Another problem with using fMRI and the other functional-imaging methods available, Koch said in Crick's office, is that "you're looking at blood activity over very long timescales, like seconds, while the thing that determines our minds are really neurons, nerve cells, and they switch at the millisecond timescale, at the thousandth-of-a-second timescale."

And so, said Crick, "what we want to do is see more people looking at neurons." In his opinion, today's consciousness researchers are making the same mistake geneticists did before his and Watson's discovery: trying to work on the problem at a macroscopic scale when the answer is more likely to come from characterizing the microscopic building blocks.

Nearing the end of his career and recognizing he wasn't equipped to address that problem himself, Crick had devoted a big part of his work after 1976 to publicizing the possibility of and need for a scientific and cell-based study of the basis of human consciousness. As part of that task, he read voraciously on the subject and conferred with those engaged in both the psychological and philosophic work on consciousness, as well as the few engaged in cellular consciousness research. He and Koch had published a number of papers attempting to synthesize the information from those different fields. When I met with them, one such article had come out recently.

"Now, did Christof show you the paper we published earlier this year?" Crick asked. It had appeared in the journal *Nature Neuroscience*, and the two hoped it would serve not only as an encouragement to neurobiologists to get in on the consciousness game, but also as a kind of plan of attack for them to do so. "Because we haven't got a lot to add to that—it's just a matter of filling it out for you."

The truth is—and Crick well knew it—that filling out the sketch they provided in that paper, titled "A Framework for Consciousness," would easily take the rest of his life and mine, and likely much longer. The article laid out in broad strokes what is known or hypothesized about the neural basis of consciousness, as well as Crick and Koch's ideas on how to tackle the problem scientifically. As Crick said regarding his astonishing hypothesis, "A very broad hypothesis, isn't it? It's nothing you can get your teeth into by itself." But in the *Nature Neuroscience* paper, he and Koch outlined their vision for how science might break the problem down into more tractable pieces. Their approach also advised making an end run around certain difficult aspects of it.

In introducing the subject, they wrote that "no one has produced any plausible explanation as to how the experience of the redness of red could arise from the actions of the brain." The statement is an allusion to what they and many others feel is the most difficult problem of consciousness, that of what philosophers call *qualia*, meaning, in this instance, the way it *feels* to be seeing red. As Koch told me, "Qualia are the elements of consciousness: the texture, the feel, the pain, the pleasure."

Qualia, many believe, are what separate us as conscious beings, who can sense and experience the world around us, from other entities that gather information from the world but don't feel anything as they do. Presumably, a camera does not have the experience of red, although it does have a method of detecting red. Plants also have detectors—anyone who has ever watched a sunflower blossom swing around to follow the sun knows they must. But if you don't believe that plants are conscious (which most of us don't, feeling no qualms about uprooting and then crunching into a carrot), you have to figure sunflowers don't have the qualia associated with the sun: what we would call warmth, yellowness, brightness, pleasure. If they did, how could we justify ending their lives by lopping off their heads and plunking them in vases for our own pleasure? An enormous question that must be answered by scientists studying consciousness is what exactly experience is and how we can have it and other living creatures don't.

Or maybe it doesn't have to be answered, at least not yet. "It appears fruitless to approach this problem head-on," Crick and Koch write in their paper, arguing that certain philosophic questions arising from the astonishing hypothesis—what consciousness is and how something so intangible, inexplicable, and undefinable can arise from the tangible, explicable, and definable matter we are made of—ought to be ignored for the moment. Until we understand exactly which cells are sufficient for consciousness, or for a particular conscious perception, they argue, we have no way of understanding the nature of, or how they achieve, that remarkable state. As Crick said to me in his office, "The whole point of our approach is to leave that question on one side—that *is* our approach—and try and find something manageable that you can do science on."

Their framework for attacking the problem consists of ten items. In the first, they advocate considering the front of the brain as a homunculus, or little man, "looking at" the back of the brain and the sensory input that arrives there first. "In general, if you have damage to the back of the brain, you don't see things or hear things or feel things," Crick said, whereas, "if you have damage to the front of the brain, you alter your character. That's a very broad—a very broad—generalization, but it gives you a general impression of what's going on." For the most part, the front of the brain puts together information brought to the back of the brain by the nerve tracts from the sensory organs. While the back of the brain does some initial processing of information from the eyes, for instance, most evidence shows that it is the front of the brain that creates meaning from that information, much as you put together images you see on your TV screen and make meaning from them.

In the second point in their paper, Crick and Koch remind their readers of the surprising fact that most ("the vast majority," Koch says) of what happens in our brains is unconscious. They call such activity "cortical reflexes" or "zombie modes" and point out that they are faster, as far as we can tell, than the conscious modes of our brains. "Take tennis," Koch offered as an example of zombie function. "If you play tennis well, most of it is totally at the zombie level. The ball approaches at high speed and your body executes the right sequence of motion to intercept the ball with your racket and return it. There is almost no delay between sensing the ball and reacting to it. It's all smooth motion, egoless, thoughtless." It is a good evolutionary strategy, he and Crick note, to have some fast, stereotyped reactions and processes in addition to a slower, integrative function like consciousness. With such a schema, consciousness can react to new and evolutionarily unanticipated circumstances while not having to dirty its hands with the mundane work of survival, which it can leave to the zombie modes.

These zombie modes can be surprising in the extent to which they can, unbeknownst to us, influence our behavior. One example the two gave was of patients who are blind on one side owing to brain damage (rather than retinal or optic-nerve damage), but who nevertheless exhibit a certain visual capacity called blindsight. "Phenomenologically they're blind," Koch said, meaning that they don't have the experience of seeing in some part of their visual field. "Yet they can do certain simple tasks." For instance, if you put a spot of light in front of a person with blindsight, placed so that it's within the area covered by the defect in their visual field, they will deny seeing the spot. "Tell them, 'Point to the light,' they say, 'Well, I don't see it,'" Koch said. But if you ask them to guess by pointing, he said, they will point and usually be correct.

This phenomenon has led scientists to conclude "that there are two—at *least* two—visual systems in your head," Koch said. "One is for conscious seeing, and one is for doing visual-motor actions. Both cases get input from the eyes, but one regulates where I put my hand." The latter, he said, needn't result in — in fact, might be encumbered by — the conscious experience of seeing. At a subsequent meeting he gave me an example, picking up his empty coffee cup, which was sitting between us. "When you grab this," he said, "it's a very sophisticated action, right? You know, you don't want to do this," he said, putting his fingers inside the cup instead of around it. "You have to judge how heavy it is, you have to sort of lift it up, in your case you have to be careful you don't spill it." (My cup was still half-full.) "It requires a lot of complicated information, but most of the information you don't have conscious access to. You just do this automatically, very quickly." So, Koch said, "The idea is that these systems that mediate this zombie behavior, these sensorimotor behaviors, they work online, in real time — they didn't evolve to deal with a delay between sensing and acting," while "the systems that seem to involve or require consciousness all have the characteristic that they can store information, at least for a short amount of time."

He and Crick theorize that "coalitions of neurons" might aid in that storage capacity, adding to the delay involved in conscious information processing, and perhaps serving as the basis of consciousness. A mention of that possibility and a call for more research on the topic serve as the third point in the pair's framework for consciousness.

It is the fourth point in their framework that has informed much of the experimental work Koch is doing. In that section of their outline, they argue that there must be "explicit representations" in our brains of things we perceive. By this they mean that if we can see a dog, whatever is happening in our brains while we're looking at the dog must be measurable and directly translatable, if we only knew what to measure and how to translate it. Thus it would be theoretically possible, by measuring the activity of neurons, to read the mind of someone looking at Fido and — simply by looking at the pattern of neuronal activity — know they were seeing a dog.

In fact, such mind reading may already be possible, at least at a crude level. Recent fMRI experiments have shown that it is possible, simply by watching subjects' brain activity, to determine the orientation of a line—ninety degrees from horizontal, sixty degrees from horizontal, and so on—at which a subject is looking. (It's important to note that this feat was possible only after having correlated each individual subject's brain activity with each line orientation. That is, the scientists had to learn what a subject's brain looked like when she viewed a line at thirty degrees from horizontal, for example, and that particular brain-activation pattern wasn't generalizable to other subjects' brains.)

It is no accident that the examples Crick and Koch use, like that of the dog or the qualia of red, are of visual perception rather than hearing, feeling, smell, or taste. Hoping to nail down, at the cellular level, what happens in our brains when we are conscious of something, the two chose to focus on the visual system, gambling that the answers for visual experience will provide a key to understanding other sorts of consciousness. They chose sight because, as Koch writes in his book *The Quest for Consciousness*, "humans are visual creatures." The fact that sight is such an enormous part of human consciousness "is reflected in the large amount of brain tissue dedicated to the analysis of images and in the importance of seeing in your daily life," he points out. "If you have a cold, for instance, your nose becomes stuffy and you lose your sense of smell, but this impairs you only mildly. A transient loss of vision, as occurs during snowblindness on the other hand, devastates you." Another reason visual perception may be the key to the scientific study of consciousness is that the large number of visual illusions that have been discovered and described make it possible to compare what happens in the brain when a stimulus is present and consciously perceived versus when it is present and not consciously perceived.* The final reason that Koch's research leans so heavily on vision is that the visual system has been extensively studied

---

* For an example of one such illusion, go to the Web content area at www.shannon moffett.com and click on the link for motion-induced blindness.

in animals; more is known about what happens to visual information in the brain than about other sensory information. Studying consciousness via vision ought, therefore, to be a bit easier than studying it via hearing or touch.

Easier doesn't mean easy, though, or even possible. Much of the study of vision has been done in monkeys, whose visual system seems fairly similar to ours. But what continues to be hard to prove is whether their consciousness is in any way similar to ours—if, indeed, it exists at all. Koch says he and most neuroscientists believe humans and monkeys have similar visual experience, given the similarity in their behaviors and visual systems. But among philosophers and even among scientists, there is still plenty of argument over whether other living creatures can be conscious. And if they can be, which are? Are bacteria? Snails? Worms? Snakes? Owls? Rats? Cats? Hogs? Dogs? There is no scientific consensus, but most agree that if any one group of nonhuman animals is conscious, it's likely to be the primates, given their close evolutionary and genetic relationship to us.

There is some convincing evidence that nonhuman primates are conscious, some of it collected by Dr. Sue Savage-Rumbaugh and her collaborators. Savage-Rumbaugh is a linguist at Georgia State University who studies animal consciousness using bonobos, one of the four species of great apes. She and her colleagues have taught bonobos to communicate with humans using a keyboard with pictures representing nouns and verbs. Using that keyboard, her bonobos seem to be able to put together rudimentary sentences, communicating ideas beyond the simple desire for food.

They can also understand verbal instructions. For instance, the bonobo Kanzi, one of the most advanced apes (by human standards, at least) ever studied, seems to have picked up an understanding of language while very young simply by overhearing the training of another bonobo, his foster mother. According to Savage-Rumbaugh, he can understand and carry out the instructions in the sentence "Go wash the potatoes, cut them up, and put them in a pot on the stove," even if he has never heard that sentence before.* Apparently, like a human's, his understanding of the meaning of verbs, nouns, and the grammatic structure of language allows him to parse and understand brand new sentences. Kanzi's half sister, Panbanisha, whose command of language exceeds Kanzi's, has apparently used her language keyboard to communicate history to her trainers—for instance, of a fight that happened between two other bonobos—hours after the events she related have happened. Such communicating of past events is one of the hallmarks of what we think of as human consciousness. Another is possession of something called "theory of mind."

A part of normal adult human consciousness is our understanding that others may have goals, desires, and beliefs separate from our own. This attribution of a separate consciousness to others is known as theory of mind. Human children don't develop a theory of mind before the age of around four and a half years old. Savage-Rumbaugh has an astonishing video showing a bonobo exhibiting what may be a theory of mind. In it, she, Panbanisha, and a "visitor" are in Panbanisha's enclosure. The visitor gives a bag of M&M's to Savage-Rumbaugh, who, in sight of her and Panbanisha, puts them in a red plastic lunch box and says to the visitor, "OK, I'm putting your M&M's right here, in this lunch box." The visitor then leaves, at which point Savage-Rumbaugh beckons to Panbanisha and opens the lunch box with her, taking the M&M's out and replacing them with pine branches. She then hides the M&M's in Panbanisha's backpack. When the visitor returns, purportedly looking for her M&M's, Panbanisha tosses a net lying on the floor of her enclosure over her own face, as if to hide it from the visitor, and falls to the floor with what can only be described as a look of merriment on her face. When asked where the

---

* I have seen a videotape of Kanzi following those instructions, although I have no way of knowing if it was the first time he'd heard the sentence.

visitor thinks the M&M's are, Panbanisha pushes the symbol for "lunch box."*

That scenario was modeled after a similar psychological test done with children, in whom it is used to diagnose certain developmental disorders, such as autism. A child younger than four or five years old (or later, in the setting of autism) usually can't grasp that anyone might hold beliefs different from her own. When asked where the visitor thought the M&M's were, a young child would have answered "in the backpack," as that's where she herself knew the candy to be. Kanzi and Panbanisha, on the other hand, seem to have developed a theory of mind and seem able to use language—not simply memorized phrases but the complex and flexible syntax of actual language—to communicate. By many scholars' criteria, those findings, if accurate, are good evidence that bonobos are conscious beings in the way that we are.

There are, of course, those who doubt Savage-Rumbaugh's data, or who argue that Kanzi's and other apes' ability to use language is either (a) not really an ability to use true language at all (notable among these is the philosopher and linguist Noam Chomsky) or (b) not evidence of consciousness at all. And so the fact remains that the only group we know for sure is conscious is humans, and ideally we would like to study consciousness in them. That, Crick and Koch explained, is exactly what Koch is doing at Caltech, where he is experimenting with human neurons in vivo.

WHILE KOCH BRIEFLY described his research as we sat in Crick's office, it wasn't until a few weeks later when I visited him at his lab in a bougainvillea-wrapped Spanish-style building on Caltech's Pasadena campus that I began to understand it. The lab is known from within as

---

* To see the video of Panbanisha, go to the Web content area at www.shannon moffett.com and click on the Panbanisha link.

the K-Lab, and Koch himself is known there as "Our Glorious Leader," or so says its student-written phone directory. The halls of the lab are decorated with the standard academic posters for presentation at scientific conferences ("Channel Noise in Excitable Neuronal Membranes," for example), but also with more whimsical artifacts of Koch's interests. There is a picture of a neuron styled to look like the map of a city, with cars driving along the cell's axon and airplanes parked on some of its dendrites, as well as a cartoon showing little white-coated scientists sitting inside a neuron, catching neurotransmitters in butterfly nets and burlap sacks and examining them in wonder. There is also a picture of two rock climbers rappelling down a sheer red cliff face. They are outlined against a blue sky in which float a few wisps of cloud through which a glimpse of earth is visible, apparently thousands of feet below. One of the climbers—long limbed and taut muscled—could be Koch; there's a thought bubble over his head that reads, "I wonder what chemical in my brain makes me go to such heights in search of pleasure."

The door to Koch's office says his name in colored wooden letters clearly designed with a child's bedroom in mind. It was closed when I arrived, and his secretary, Candi, who was wearing an appropriately pink-and-white-striped shirt, told me he hadn't arrived yet. He showed up moments later, his hair now the copper of a new penny, and said, "Hello, hello, let me just check one thing and I'll be right with you," as he breezed by into his office.

"He's always like this," Candi said. Peering in after him, I could see a room furnished predominantly in purple and teal, with a phrenology bust atop a bank of file cabinets, and a globe of Mars ("one of the few Mars globes on the planet," Koch told me later) hanging from the ceiling. In a moment he emerged and took me upstairs to buy a cup of coffee before we settled on a bench outside his building, by a fountain whose arched jets made a tunnel beneath the brilliant blue Southern California sky.

We began by talking about rock climbing, which seems to serve Koch as an ongoing study of the coordinated use of both conscious and zombie modes of his brain. "It's this perfect fusion of intellect and mind and body," he said. "You never feel as alive as if you are somewhere suspended five hundred foot up on a wall and there's the wind howling and you look down and you see these little people there, and it's just you and the rope and your partner and the blue sky and the sun. YEEE-OOOOOO!" He gave a piercing cry of pure delight that resounded off the walls of the academic buildings around us. "It feels— there's really nothing like it. And then you make it to the top and— it's like making love to a woman for twelve hours, I mean it's very, very intense." Koch is scarcely less enthusiastic about his work in the lab, which he turned to next. "There's, with maybe one or two exceptions," he said, "nobody else on the planet who records directly from neurons in humans."

Nobody else does it because such experiments require inserting electrodes into a person's brain, meaning Koch can't just offer a Jamba Juice gift certificate and watch the undergraduates roll up to his door volunteering to serve as subjects, as he could with an imaging study. And in fact, at any level of recompense, internal review boards, the university committees that approve study designs, consider voluntary craniotomies unethical, citing the risks to the individual from infection or accidental brain damage.*

---

* Both Crick and Koch consider this stance curious. Crick has pointed out that in the U.S. we can join the military and risk death to serve our country, but there is no way to volunteer for invasive experiments in service to mankind. When I asked, both of them claimed they would volunteer themselves if they could. "Oh, yes, certainly I would," Crick said, "because I think the information is extremely valuable, and I think the risks are rather small."

Koch said he wouldn't mind: "You have to drill a little hole," he said, "a tiny burr hole that's two millimeters. That's the only thing that's painful, but you give local anesthetic." But then he added, "You know, I wouldn't mind maybe having *one* burr hole." But some studies require at least two, and "my wife has said she'll probably divorce me before I do that."

Some people, however, need to have electrodes implanted in their brains for medical reasons, and Koch's study, performed in collaboration with Dr. Itzhak Fried, is with those patients. Fried is a neurosurgeon and the director of epilepsy surgery at the UCLA School of Medicine. As William Scoville did with HM, Fried occasionally finds it hard to discover where exactly in his patients' brains their seizures are beginning. It's important — as Scoville learned — to locate the seizure focus as precisely as possible, allowing removal of the smallest bit of brain necessary to alleviate the seizures while causing the least collateral damage. In order to do that, Fried drills holes in his patients' skulls and places electrodes on the surface of — and sometimes inside — their brains. The electrodes are usually located in the medial temporal lobe, some in the hippocampus, some in the amygdala of his patients, who spend a couple of days in the hospital afterward, just hanging out and waiting to have a seizure. When they do, Fried can localize it by reading the signals from the implanted electrodes. In the meantime, the patients are in the hospital, electrodes in their brains, awake and conscious and without anything else to do, making them perfect subjects for Koch's research.

While the electrodes surgeons use to track seizures are too big to catch a signal from a single neuron, those Fried uses have a hollow core, allowing skinnier microelectrodes to be threaded through them and situated, as Koch says, "close enough to one neuron or two neurons that you can hear them over the din created by all the other neurons." The brain is "a very noisy place, electrically speaking," he explained as we sipped our coffee outside his lab. "You hear the faint echo of the activity of thousands of neurons, most of which you can't distinguish. But if you're very close to one neuron, much closer to one neuron than to other neurons, you can mainly listen to that neuron."

Koch's experiment, which had been going on for about four years at the time we spoke, consists of listening to those single neurons while showing Dr. Fried's patients images of familiar objects and people. About once a month a patient is scheduled for this neuro-surgical procedure and agrees to participate in the study. "When it happens, it's very absorbing," Koch said. "I mean, the two people from my lab who are down there, they spend, like, essentially four days down in the clinic, taking the data, and then spending the next three weeks till the next patient analyzing it."* What they are looking for in that analysis are neurons that fire only during the conscious visual perception of some objects and not others, neurons that might be part of the neural correlates of consciousness for which he is hunting.

The problem is, no one knows how many neurons might be expected to be part of the NCC. One possibility was put forward in 1969 by Dr. Jerome Lettvin, a neurophysiologist at MIT, who is credited with first using the phrase *grandmother cells*. The term, Koch explained, refers to the possibility that "for every percept, like the percept of your grandmother," there is "a group of neurons that specifically only fires for your grandmother." Most scientists are skeptical of that theory, pointing out, as Koch put it, that "there are a gazillion number of concepts and ideas that I could have, and there aren't enough neurons" to allow such specificity. And so, he said, "people don't like it, and they prefer the alternative, which is population coding, that you have a very large set of neurons responding—in different ways—to distinct objects out there in the world; they fire in one way to Grandma, in another way to Grandpa, and in a third manner to other aged relatives." The idea that particular cells exclusively represent a person or object is out of favor.

---

* One of the facts of academic life is that much of the work "done" by the heads of university laboratories is really done by their graduate students and postdoctoral fellows, who don't always get the recognition they deserve, reflecting a traditional prejudice against junior researchers. In these studies, the people who actually went to the UCLA Hospital and spent hours interviewing the subjects and then even more hours working with the raw data were Koch's graduate student Leila Reddy and postdoctoral fellow Dr. Rodrigo Quian-Quiroga.

Nevertheless, Fried and Koch may have found some such cells in their experiments recording from single neurons. "We have neurons," Koch told me, "that seem to respond very specifically, there's no question about it," to images of particular things and not others. For example, Gabriel Kreiman, at the time a graduate student in Koch's lab, found "one neuron that only responds to three very different pictures of Bill Clinton: a color portrait, a pencil drawing, and a portrait with him and two others—his wife and somebody else," he said. "The images couldn't be more different at the pixel level, but the neuron responds very strongly to all of them." The neuron was not active at baseline, when its owner wasn't being shown a picture, and it did not respond to images of other men, other famous people, animals, objects, or landmarks.

"Now I cannot exclude," Koch said, "that it might respond to yet another Southern Baptist politician, because we only had half an hour to record from, and you know, in that time you can only show so many images."

Because the experiments took place in the brief period during which the subjects had electrodes implanted before surgery, Koch's team also wasn't able to show the patient whose neuron responded to the pictures of Clinton other things that might logically excite that neuron if it were indeed part of the neural correlate of the conscious idea of Bill Clinton—the written words *Bill Clinton*, for example, or photos of Monica Lewinsky, or a recording of Clinton's voice. "Until recently," Koch told me, "we had the following problem: we went in the clinic, we showed the patient blindly hundred images, we recorded everything, we went off-line. It took us two weeks to analyze the data."

That analysis might show, for instance, as it did in one of Koch's subjects, that they had found a neuron that seemed to respond only to photos of the Beatles. But by the time they had discovered which neuron responded to which class of images, the patient had already had the electrodes removed and undergone the surgery. So it was impossible to do the obvious follow-up experiments — showing individual pictures of the faces of John, Paul, George, and Ringo, for instance, or of Yoko's face; showing a picture of the *White Album;* playing the *White Album;* showing pictures of the Monkees.

However, Koch's group had recently figured out a way to streamline their analysis so that follow-up experiments with the same subjects are possible. Now, he told me, "we can do what's called a.m./p.m. experiments. We test patients in the morning, we read out data from sixty-four electrodes, we can do a very quick analysis for the next two hours, and then we can come and say, 'OK, these neurons seem to respond very specifically.' For example, last time we had neurons that responded to the Tower of Pisa, and to Jennifer Aniston. And then we can come back in the afternoon and say, 'OK, let's show now thirty different pictures of Jennifer Aniston.'"

Probably the biggest problem with Fried's and Koch's results is that even if we do have grandmother cells, it's hard to believe his method would have found any. There are roughly a hundred billion neurons in the human brain. The images Koch and his collaborators choose to show to patients are images of well-known things and people, and presumably there would be more than one neuron dedicated to representing them in our brains, but still, "it's very unlikely to find these neurons, right?" Koch said when I broached the subject. "Yeah. That's what bothers me. Everybody asks us, and I don't know."

Calculating the odds of finding, by chance, a neuron representing one of the gazillion things there are in the world, even if a few thousand such neurons existed in a single brain, is not an easy statistical problem. Usually, scientists try to calculate the likelihood that their results, which may appear to be meaningful evidence of a trend, are based on chance alone. It's important to make such calculations because, by necessity, science is usually done on a sample of a population rather than on the whole of that population. Whether you're studying the behavior of neurons or songbirds or people or the stock market, you're rarely going to be taking measurements from each and every member of the population under study. So when you make a generalization from the sample you study to the population at large, there is a chance — bigger or smaller depending on factors like the size of your sample compared to the size of the population as a whole, how well you controlled for other variables, and so forth — that the trend or trait you observed is characteristic only of that sample and not of the population at large.

Because Koch's experiments deal with a population of people, a population of neurons, and a population of familiar objects and people, and because his samples are so small compared to the total population of any of those, figuring out how to statistically analyze his data is close to impossible. After my talk with Koch in Pasadena, I spoke with Dr. Paul Switzer, a professor of statistics at Stanford. Over a pitcher of beer at the Stanford Coffee House, I described Koch's experiments to Switzer and asked him what he thought the odds are that Koch has actually found a Bill Clinton neuron or a Beatles neuron, given the arbitrary nature of his selection of both neurons and images. Switzer thought for a moment, took a sip of beer, and leaned back in his chair. "Remote," he said.

Switzer acknowledged that even he doesn't really know how to approach the problem, although he, like Koch, had plenty of ideas for follow-up experiments that might clarify the picture a bit. Koch himself is acutely aware of the difficulty of interpreting his data. And yet, "All I can tell you, we find these neurons, no question about it," he said.

Nevertheless, the first papers Koch and Fried published on the topic don't focus on the highly selective nature of the neurons they've found. Instead, one reports the fact that when they showed a subject a picture and then had her close her eyes and *imagine* that picture, a neuron that fired selectively when she actually saw the image also fired when she called it up in her "mind's eye." This finding in itself was interesting but not entirely surprising, as fMRI studies have shown that the same areas of the brain are activated when a subject is imagining a motor task, like tapping her fingers, as when she's actually performing it. But it did serve as evidence that they had actually come upon a cell having something to do with the *conscious* experience of a visual image, rather than just a cell at a low (and unconscious) level of visual processing.

Another paper Fried and Koch published presents more evidence that the neurons they found did, in fact, fire in correlation with conscious experience. The experiments for that paper involved making use of something called flash suppression. It has long been known that, given the same visual information, our conscious experience of that visual information may differ—from one person to another, of course, but even an individual will make different meanings at different times out of the same visual information. A classic example is the Necker cube:

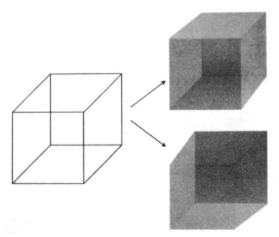

Because it's a two-dimensional drawing, it can only *represent* depth, but it does a good job of tricking you into seeing a three-dimensional object. If you look long enough, though, you can experience what happens as your mind tries to make sense of the two-dimensional lines on the page. When you first look at the drawing, it may appear to be a cube receding back into the page at an upward slant from the face "closest" to you. But if you look at it steadily for a few seconds, it will switch, appearing to recede with a downward slant. If you keep looking at the picture, your experience will shift back and forth between these two possible meanings of the representation, even though all the while the same information has been presented to your retina. Nothing about the drawing changes, but your conscious experience of it does. What happens in your brain during that switch from one experience to the other is something scientists studying consciousness would like to know.

A similar switch between two possible conscious experiences of the same retinal input occurs with binocular rivalry. In that phenomenon, hard to demonstrate without special equipment, two different images are presented, one to each eye, without letting one eye see what the other does. The images have to be carefully balanced for luminance and other properties, but when they are, people don't see a blend of the two images, and they don't see just one of the images and completely ignore the other. As with the Necker cube, a subject presented with a different image in each eye will "see"—where *see* means "have a visual experience of"—first one of the images and then the other.

If, for example, as I once saw demonstrated by a researcher at a consciousness conference, you are presented with an image of Darth Vader in one eye and of Yoda in the other, there will be what he characterized as a battle between Good and Evil in your own brain, with each side alternately gaining the upper hand. You don't experience the battle, but you do experience the results, alternately seeing the elderly green Jedi knight and the black-helmeted Dark Lord of the Sith.

Your awareness of each of the pictures alternates, that is, if the pictures are presented at the same time. But if you've been looking with your right eye at a picture of Yoda and with the left eye at nothing, just a quick flash of a picture of Darth Vader in your left eye is enough to tip the battle to the dark side, and you'll be conscious of seeing the picture of Darth Vader. That phenomenon is called flash suppression and was used by Koch's lab in one of the experiments they did with Fried's patients. In that study, they first showed a picture in one of a subject's eyes, then briefly flashed a different picture in the other eye, while recording activity in the neurons monitored by the microelectrodes. The instant the new picture was flashed, the subjects saw only that picture; they ceased to be aware of the first picture despite the fact that it was still there in front of one eye.

On analyzing the data, Koch's team found that neurons selective for a particular image—for instance, the image of Bill Clinton—fired steadily when that image was shown to one of a subject's eyes, but then stopped firing when a second picture was flashed in the other eye. Thus the Clintion-specific neuron stopped firing when its owner was no longer conscious of the picture of Bill Clinton. Koch sees this finding as further evidence that the neurons they have identified are, indeed, part of the neural correlates of consciousness.

If they are, how exactly those neurons correlate to conscious experience is unclear: not all the selective neurons Koch's team has found fire in a way consistent with their being grandmother cells—that is, with their being activated by only a single conscious perception. It turns out some of the cells seem to respond to categories of things, rather than to any one thing in particular: for instance, to faces, to natural scenes, to any famous person, or to animals. This finding has led Koch to dream up another experiment he'd like to do, one that relies, he said, "on the trick so beautifully exploited by Bill Newsome."

Dr. Bill Newsome is a vision researcher based at Stanford who records single-neuron responses in monkeys in experiments similar to Koch's work in humans. In the experiment Koch was referring to, Newsome trained monkeys to signal whether a group of moving dots on a computer screen were moving to the left or to the right. By measuring from electrodes implanted in a monkey's brain, he was able to find small clusters of neurons active only when the monkey signaled the dots were moving to the left. He also found neurons active only when the monkey thought the dots were moving to the right.

Newsome then made it harder to tell which direction the dots were moving in by introducing other randomly moving dots as interference.* He added more and more interference until there came a point where the monkey was apparently just guessing. About 50 percent of the time it would guess the dots were moving to the right, and 50 percent of the time it would guess they were moving to the left; but the guesses had no apparent relation to which way the dots were actually moving. Newsome found, however, that he could influence the monkey's guesses using the electrodes implanted in its brain. Instead of using them to record neuronal activity, he sent electricity through them. That current activated the neurons at the electrode's tip. If those neurons had previously fired when the monkey signaled the dots were moving to the left, stimulating them made the monkey tend to guess the dots were moving to the left. If Newsome sent electricity through electrodes implanted near the motion-to-the-right neurons, the monkey would tend to guess the dots were moving to the right.

Koch would like to adapt Newsome's experiment for use with his human subjects. Once he's identified a cluster of neurons that selectively fire when a subject is shown pictures of animals, Koch said he'd then show pictures of animals and cars morphed together to varying degrees. "I show you many pictures between the animal and the car and you could say, 'OK, it's basically an animal,'" he said. "And then we're adding more and more of a car; at some point you say, 'Well, I don't know. Is it an animal or a car?'"

---

* Newsome has put examples of the random-dot stimuli the monkeys are shown on his Web site. You can link to them from the Web content area of www.shannon moffett.com.

Imagine, he said, "you're at this middle point where you could say, 'Well, it's either a car or an animal.' Now inject current." If the surgeon sent current through the implanted electrodes, the electrodes would excite nearby neurons, and in theory, that excitation would be accompanied by whatever conscious perception those neurons' firing usually elicits. But would it work in practice? "Is it now possible," Koch asked, "to change the percept of the person?" No one knows.

If all this talk of zapping the brain sounds frightening, it's helpful to remember that the current Koch dreams of using is only about ten microamps, or about a millionth of that supplied by a wall socket. Surgeons routinely stimulate patients' brains with such currents when mapping out functional areas of the brain to plan the least destructive path for their operations.

What's really unsettling—though it is of course a logical corollary to Crick's astonishing hypothesis—is the idea that Koch might be able to change his subjects' experience by stimulating their brains. That such stimuli can and do change people's behavior and feelings has been shown, Koch tells me. Electrical current applied directly to the brain can cause a patient to stop speaking, to move her arms or legs, to hear a particular piece of music, to feel an emotion. He described a patient of Fried's, a sixteen-year-old epileptic. While mapping her brain preparatory to removing the locus of her seizures, Fried found there was a particular spot in her brain that, when stimulated with a weak current, caused her to smile. A stronger current applied to the area induced what he called in his paper describing her case "a robust contagious laughter."

Both the smiling and the laughter were accompanied by a feeling of mirth and amusement, according to the patient. She had been asked to perform several different kinds of tasks—naming objects, tapping her fingers, reading aloud. Fried's team stimulated the laughter-provoking part of her brain as she performed each of the tasks. Each time, they asked her what had made her laugh, and each time, she gave a different answer based on what she was doing at the moment. "Thus," as Fried wrote in his description of the phenomenon, her "laughter was attributed to the particular object seen during naming ('the horse is funny'), to the particular content of a paragraph during reading, or to persons present in the room while the patient performed a finger apposition task ('you guys are just so funny . . . standing around')."

According to Koch, Fried has also found areas in the brain that when stimulated result in a patient's experiencing a strong memory or hallucination.

Koch and Fried's work so far is purely theoretical, but others are trying to put findings like Fried's to practical use. "If you are blind, if you lose your retina," said Koch, "there are people trying to directly stimulate with electrodes the back of your brain, the visual part." Such stimulation, based on light patterns picked up by electronic sensors, could essentially replace the retina and optic nerve with man-made hardware. So far, the implants have elicited only phosphenes (the little flashes of light you see when you close your eyes), but some researchers claim that in some cases patients implanted with such electrodes can navigate based on the shapes the phosphenes outline.

SOME OF THE DIFFICULTY in developing functional vision prostheses may be due to what Crick and Koch call the complex and "layered" nature of consciousness. In Crick's office, after Koch had briefly outlined the work he would later detail for me at Caltech, we discussed the fifth of the ten points in their framework for studying consciousness. Crick explained a concept they have labeled "higher levels first" by noting that if we see a flash of light or movement, we may well be aware that something happened before we are aware of what, exactly. Often the information required to figure out what happened has already been transmitted to our brains by, in the case of the visual system, our eyes and optic nerves. But we don't immediately become aware of everything our eyes send to our brains; rather, the overall gist of a scene arrives first in our consciousness, followed by the specifics.

If there is a disruption in processing between the presentation of the visual scene and our awareness of its details, we may never become aware of the details. One example of such a disruption is visual masking, which I saw demonstrated at a conference by Dr. Vince Di Lollo, a psychologist at the University of British Columbia in Vancouver. The example he showed consisted first of a fixation point, a cross that appeared a moment before anything else. He told his audience to look at the cross. A moment later, a field of several shapes—triangles, circles, diamonds, and so on—flashed on the screen. One of the shapes was highlighted by a square of four dots surrounding it, like this:

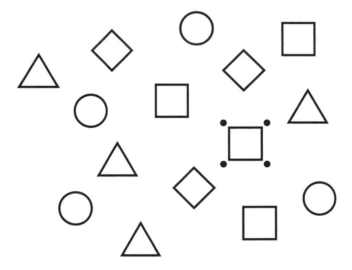

The entire field of shapes was flashed for only ten milliseconds—a hundredth of a second—but it was possible to identify the shape outlined by the four dots, even in that brief instant. That is, until Di Lollo showed the whole series again, this time leaving the four dots surrounding the shape in place after the shape itself disappeared. The result of that simple change was that we could no longer identify which shape had been outlined by the four dots. It was surprising and infuriating. I'd been able to see that there was a shape and had the sense that I could identify it, but when I tried to, I couldn't.*

This particular version of masking is called backward masking, because after a first stimulus is shown, a subsequent stimulus masks the first from conscious perception; but there are examples of forward masking and simultaneous masking as well, many of which involve, as Koch and Crick describe in their paper, a sensation of "something" happening that is unidentifiable. As with other consciously unperceived phenomena described here, it turns out that the idea of the shape doesn't vanish without a trace; experiments have shown that subjects shown such masked shapes and then asked to guess which shape was masked will guess much more accurately than could be expected if their guesses were guided only by chance.

Not surprisingly, Crick and Koch believe the key to understanding such mysteries lies in studying individual neurons. Until we understand the interactions of one neuron with another, they argue in the sixth point in their framework, we are going to have a hard time understanding the neural basis of consciousness or any complicated brain processes. Returning to the million neurons in his grain-of-rice-size piece of cortex, Koch said, "They're all very, very different. They're all highly distinct, and they're heterogeneous, and we really need to understand—"

Crick, who seems to have acted as a curb to Koch's more extravagant nature, cut in to say drily, "There are many different types. I'm not sure they're all highly distinct."

Koch ceded the point but went on to say that even if there are only a hundred different neuron types, "they're not just in a soup. They all have very specific interactions." In his opinion and in Crick's, understanding those interactions and knowing what makes one group of cells different from another might be the key to understanding how our minds arise from our brains.

* For a demonstration of backward masking, visit the Web content area of www
   .shannonmoffett.com.

At that point, Odile appeared at the door to Crick's study to ask if we were ready for lunch. Crick assured her we would be soon, and then the two launched into the seventh point in their framework, of which "the basic idea," Crick said, "is that consciousness is not a continuous stream, but it's a series of short batches." So what Koch calls the "movie in your brain" of visual perception may, like a movie, actually consist of rapidly successive still snapshots, with motion "painted on" over them.

Although our consciousness feels to us as continuous and unified as a movie, there is evidence it is in fact spliced together from scraps by our brains. For example: "You should realize," Crick said to me, that "motion and position are signaled differently. And the easiest way to learn that is the so-called waterfall effect." Known less romantically as the motion aftereffect, the phenomenon can be experienced by first staring continuously at something characterized by movement in a single direction, such as a waterfall. Afterward, if you divert your eyes to stationary objects (rocks beside the waterfall, for instance), they will appear to move upward. "They don't change position," Crick said, "but they appear to be moving."* From animal studies and functional imaging in humans, it appears the part of the brain where the clusters for movement-to-the-left or movement-to-the-right are located in Newsome's monkeys—the area known as V5 or MT—is also activated when people perceive motion that isn't there, as they do momentarily after having gazed at a waterfall.†

---

* A demo of the waterfall effect can be found in the Web content area at www.shannonmoffett.com. Try looking at your own hand after looking at the waterfall, too.

† Presumably, although this is still under study, the perception of stillness is achieved by a kind of tug-of-war between neurons for motion-to-the-left and those for motion-to-the-right, as well as those for motion-up and motion-down. When an object isn't moving, the tugs-of-war are at a draw. The theory is that as we look at the waterfall, the neurons for motion-down are being so continuously stimulated that they adapt to fire less strongly, so when you then look at a static object, they can't fire strongly enough to counteract the motion-up neurons.

Crick also described the case of a woman who'd been rendered motion-blind by a stroke. She apparently experienced the world as if it were a movie mismatched with its audiotrack. If she began a conversation with a man standing in front of her, she couldn't watch his lips move. If he moved around behind her, for a moment she would continue to experience him visually in front of her, although she could hear his change in position by following his voice. Every once in a while, she'd experience a new visual snapshot, which she could compare to her memory of the last. "She could *infer* motion, but she never saw motion," Crick said. "The brain damage had knocked out her motion sensor."

Koch mentioned similar evidence supporting the idea that consciousness only appears continuous to us. He and Crick had recently met with Dr. Oliver Sacks, a neurologist and the author of, among other books, *The Man Who Mistook His Wife for a Hat,* which describes cases of consciousness-altering brain damage he's seen in his career. Sacks has decribed patients, Koch told me, who experience something Sacks calls "cinematographic vision" following brain damage. It's a condition some migraineurs also suffer from, although in them it is transient (Sacks himself has experienced it during migraines). People with the condition describe seeing the world as if it were a movie run at a very slow speed. "So instead of seeing smooth motion you actually see the individual frames," Koch explained, experiencing "what you might see in a disco," where strobe lights make it impossible to see people dancing but allow rapidly successive glimpses of them in different positions, from which motion can be deduced.

These cases in which perception of motion has been selectively removed from consciousness, along with other similar evidence, have led Crick and Koch to believe that, as with a movie, our experience of consciousness as an uninterrupted stream has more to do with the rate at which our consciousness samples the information available to it than with any true continuity of those bits of information. They think it likely that temporal "smearing" in that sampling (meaning we hang on to one perceptual snapshot long enough that it overlaps the next), along with our capacity for experiencing "motion" independent of actual position change, work together to create the sense of seamlessness inherent to normal consciousness.

"When you have, let's say, a red Ferrari," Koch said, "you have this sound, this unique low-frequency rumble, and you see red and you see motion—well, so really there are three things: there's this sound, the color, the motion. Do you really experience them at the same time? Now, at the perceptual timescale, sure." But it's possible, he said—and some recent data support this idea—that the information you perceive as happening at the same time is really reaching your brain at different times. "So you have activity in the brain that evolves continuously," he said. But their hypothesis is that some coalitions of neurons might work in a more discrete way, sampling information from the continuously evolving neurons moment by moment and creating sequential conscious snapshots out of that information. And perhaps, said Koch, "those are the ones that underlie our perception of the world."

"If we could establish that, that would be a step forward," Crick said. "But of course it may not be right."

Those coalitions of neurons are the subject of the eighth and ninth items in his and Koch's framework for consciousness. In the eighth, they point out that either your attention can be grabbed or you can focus it consciously (with the latter process being slower) and argue that attention probably acts by affecting the competition among "rival coalitions" fighting to reach the threshold we call consciousness. In their ninth point, the two briefly discuss synchronized firing of neurons, which they had at one time hypothesized might be the sole basis of the NCC. That is, if a set of neurons were firing in synchrony, you would be conscious of whatever they represented—the throbbing of a headache or the white of the wall in front of you or the sound of a Mozart sonata. They no longer think synchronized firing alone is sufficient to be the NCC, but still maintain that it, like attention, might help give a boost to a coalition contesting for consciousness.

Finally, in the last point of their framework, the two take a stab at "meaning," a real problem for neuroscientists, as it's hard to quantify and no one is quite sure what meaning means. As Koch now said to me, "Red for you *means* all sorts of things, right? It means the clothes you wear"—I was, in fact, wearing a red shirt with white polka dots that day—"and the 'little red book' of Mao, and the red sunset, and all sorts of other red things. And the same thing with blue or pleasure or the salty texture of potato chips or whatever. These are all meaningful states, and so the question is, How do these states acquire meaning?"

Crick pointed out that even if Koch is able to identify which neurons fire with the conscious experience of red, we still won't necessarily understand how the brain knows what that firing represents. Their hunch, which they describe in their framework, is that meaning may rest in what they call the "penumbra" of the neurons firing with conscious experience. They define the penumbra as the set of all neurons responding in some way to the firing of the neurons correlated with the consciousness of redness. And they argue that whether or not the penumbra is part of the NCC proper at the moment you become conscious of redness, the penumbra—the neurons representing valentines, blood, William Carlos Williams's wheelbarrow, Koch's Ferrari—may give meaning to the percept and somehow help it either achieve or maintain its conscious status.

ABOUT AN HOUR after Odile had appeared at the door of Crick's study to say that lunch was ready, we joined her at a table off the kitchen. The talk turned less scientific, or at least less neuroscientific, when I asked Crick and Odile how they met.

"Well, I was in the Wrens, which was the equivalent of the WAVs here," Odile said. "And I was translating—"

"In the London headquarters," Crick cut in.

"Yes. Boring documents about torpedoes and mines, from German to English. And one evening—I was sharing an apartment with another friend from art school—"

"A girlfriend," Crick said.

"Yes, a girlfriend. And then we—I happened to go into the office where the main part of the department of torpedoes and mines was—"

"Where I wasn't working, but I was visiting." Crick's office at the time was located in Portsmouth. This would have been in 1944, they decided.

"So I was sitting—I had a little office there—"

"Upstairs—"

"Yes. And I was translating these documents, day after day, not very interesting."

"So you understood all these very complicated German technical terms?" Koch asked.

"Ye-es," Odile said.

"No," Crick said.

"Well, I had a dictionary to help me."

"She really didn't understand electricity at all," Crick said fondly.

"Well, I translated the words that I saw. They must be terrible. I expect it's been—I *hope* it's been thrown out."

"I'll tell you my electricity story later," Crick said. "But go on, finish the story, darling—this is taking forever."

"OK. Well, I went down—I always used to go and see the people in the department, which were all men, and just say good-bye."

"This department had a big office," Crick said.

"Yes, a small office," Odile said.

"Downstairs."

"Of about four or five naval officers. And I opened the door, and out came this very strange-looking man, with sort of stoopy shoulders and a kind of very scruffy raincoat on. And I was holding one of my bags of brussels sprouts, which I was taking home to cook, and the bottom fell out of the bag. So he picked them all up and said, 'Come out to dinner.'" She stopped to laugh. "And I said, 'Oh, no, I've got to go home and cook supper.' I thought, 'Well, what a dangerous man,' you know, how *fast*," she said, still laughing.

"But I'd found out where she was working, so next time I came, I could go up and say hello to her, you see," Crick said. "That was a quite clever thing to do, to find out."

"So you did not go out, you did not have dinner that time?" Koch asked.

"No, but later on I had lunch with him."

"That's right, that was safer," Crick said. He and Odile were married a few years later, in 1949. Shortly afterward he and Odile had a conversation about electricity, which he recounted as we ate lunch. "When we were married," he said, "in those days the electrical plugs in the wall had two things, not three—they didn't have the earth in those days." He was referring to the third prong that is now standard on electrical plugs and provides a ground. "And Odile was ironing or something like that, and she looked at it and she said, 'I suppose it has two plugs so it doesn't swivel round.'" Crick smiled and Odile laughed. "And I said 'well, that's a good explanation, but it happens not to be the correct one.' And she said, 'Don't tell me there are two wires, because look, there's only one wire.' OK, so then we had to go back and show that gosh, isn't that extraordinary, within one wire is actually two wires, you see. She was very surprised, indeed. And she says, 'Well, do you mean to say it goes down one wire and comes back the other wire?' Well, it was alternating current, but I wasn't going to fuss, and I said, 'Well, yes, that's broadly right.' 'Well, then,' she says— notice how logical it all was—'why do we pay for it?' So that was her knowledge of electricity, you see."

"You mean, because it comes back, you don't need to pay for it," Koch said.

"So heaven knows what those translations were like," Crick said.

Of course, he and Koch may easily be making an error in thinking about consciousness every bit as silly as Odile's regarding electricity. Even in writing their initial papers on DNA's structure, Crick and James Watson made assumptions that later proved erroneous — for example, that RNA probably couldn't make a double-helical structure like DNA's, which we now know it can.

"We were just too naïve at that state. I was only just beginning," Crick told me fifty years later. "We know in general what we said was on the right lines." But it turned out genetic replication is much more complicated than they realized at the time. "There's all sorts of feedbacks and networks and so on, just in a single cell," he said. "And I think the brain is going to go the same way." Regarding the neuronal organization underlying consciousness, he said, "I think when it's fully understood, it'll be seen how sophisticated and elaborate it is, and what evolution has produced." But that understanding will happen slowly. First, he predicted, "We'll get a sort of vague overall picture, and it'll gradually get more and more complicated. And hopefully at one or two points it'll get a little simpler."

I asked Crick if, this early in the search, he had a gut feeling about how and where consciousness arises from the brain, or whether the astonishing hypothesis will hold true. "We have gut feelings that local neurons matter, and how they interact globally," he said. "On the other hand, what the answer's going to be — all the experience in other biological things says that it can be right under your nose and you won't see it. That's why the subject's so difficult, because we don't know exactly what we're looking for. If we had some really good idea of what we were looking for, then it would advance much more quickly." Then he quoted the theoretical physicist Steven Weinberg: "'We do not know in advance what are the right questions to ask, and we often do not find out until we are close to the answer,'" he said. "And that's really the reply to your question."

INTERLUDE: Childhood

A month or two before you were born, most of your neurons had finished their outward journey and their axons had threaded their way through the brain to synapse with other neurons. Until then, the progenitor cells that created those neurons had remained deep inside the brain at the lining of the ventricles, steadily dividing to crank out more cells. Once that task was done, however, the progenitor cells themselves migrated a short distance outward toward the brain's surface. There they turned to producing glial cells.

Glia means "glue" in Greek, and it used to be thought that the cells, which make up about 50 percent of your brain's volume and may outnumber neurons by as much as ten to one, existed solely to hold those neurons together. That impression turned out to be false. Early in your brain's development, the radial glia—those guide-rope cells that helped neurons find their way from the inner to the outer surface of your brain—were crucial for the correct structuring of your cerebral cortex. Later, two other kinds of glia developed from the progenitor cells: astrocytes and oligodendrocytes. Astrocytes have projections known as end feet, which surround the brain's capillaries and help maintain the blood-brain barrier. Other astrocyte projections wrap around synapses to assist in neurons' reuptake of neurotransmitter molecules after they're released.

Oligodendrocytes, the other type of glial cell, are actually more like electrical tape than glue. Beginning when you were a seven- or eight-month-old fetus, each oligodendrocyte extended processes radiating out from its cell body. It used those processes to latch onto a nearby neuron's axon and wrap around it.

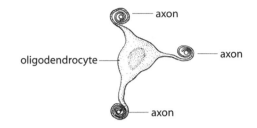

It kept wrapping and wrapping until one portion of the axon was enveloped in the multilayered coating called myelin, made up of the oligodendrocyte's cell membrane. Each oligodendrocyte might wrap several sections of one axon, or sections of several different neurons' axons. Once each of its processes has myelinated a section of axon, an oligodendrocyte simply stays put, tethered to the neurons it has wrapped. Like a neuron, an oligodendrocyte—barring injury or disease—lasts a lifetime.

Because of the fat in the oligodendrocytes' membranes, myelin is white. While the cortical gray matter composing the outer surface of the brain is made mostly of astrocytes and the unmyelinated bodies of neurons, beneath that surface is a layer of white matter, made up of millions of axons in their white myelin sheaths. Like conduit-encased cables in a house's walls, those axons carry messages to and fro, from one bit of gray matter to another.

Once they begin, oligodendrocytes myelinate axons for years. On the day you were born, when they had been at work for only a few weeks, your brain weighed a little less than a pound. By the time you were three years old, it weighed about two and a half pounds, with most of that increase due to myelination. After that and well into your childhood, myelination continued as you learned to talk, walk, tie your shoes, and read and write.

Directed thinking is not the same as thinking in a dream. We go to
sleep not for the rest but for the dream. Usually conscious life is
separate but sometimes it's the same as the dream.

—NORMAN FISCHER

4 | The Dreaming Brain

I AM FLYING DOWN the mountain in a crouch, skis under me, leaning hard and cutting my edges into a turn so that I can straighten out before hitting the black ice I know is around the bend. Last time I didn't manage it and skidded at full speed into the cliff bounding the course. I was unhurt, even after bouncing off the rock face and tumbling head over heels several times before regaining my balance, but I can't afford another delay. I'm going for speed here, trying to break my record.

This time the ice is no problem, and aside from a couple of my competitors' crashing into me (at whom I shout, "What's YOUR problem?" as I have so many times before), I make it to the bottom of the run without incident and in record time. Shaky and drenched in sweat, I pry my fingers from around the poles and step out of the bindings onto the linoleum floor of Beth Israel Deaconess Medical Center.

Later that night I'm too wired to sleep. Motion sensors are taped to my forehead and left eye, a gizmo below my chin measures muscle tension, and four electrodes glued to my scalp are tracking my brain waves. Covering the electrodes is a red bandanna, tied at the back of my head. I look like the love child of Aunt Jemima and a Borg.

When I close my eyes and try to drift off, I can still see the alpine racecourse streaming out in front of me. I float along it over and over, seeing the turns, rounding them, and flying onward. Suddenly the computer I'm plugged into says, "Wake up!" and sets me doing math problems. "353 + 412 = ?" flashes on the screen, just like that, in a horizontal line. Groggy, I punch in "567" on the keyboard. "Wrong!" says the computer, and gives me another problem, which I also get wrong. Eventually I wake up enough to answer some of the problems correctly, but it keeps throwing them at me, occasionally tossing in a subtraction problem just to screw me up. Fifteen minutes later it stops, and I can go back to sleep.

Then I am in New York City, trying to explain to my mother that we'll be meeting at Sixtieth Street, which seems like a coincidence, since sixty is five times twelve, but she shouldn't let that worry her.

Manhattan is suddenly Boston, and I am walking down Longwood Avenue, not with my mom, but with Dr. Bob Stickgold. We are tiny amid the buildings of the Longwood Medical Area, a 175-acre campus of hospitals, clinics, and research facilities that surrounds the Harvard Medical School and includes Beth Israel, where Stickgold works. In my dream, he echoes something he said to me in waking life. "One of the challenges in my life," Stickgold says, "is to be a dream researcher, which makes me one of a class of scientific flakes."

THE NEXT MORNING I wake up in Stickgold's sleep lab, remove the wires and bandanna, and walk down the hall to find Stickgold reading at his desk. Just inside the door to his office is an expanse of clinically white countertop and a sink with a high, arched spigot. On the ceiling are tracks for two nonexistent curtains to be drawn around two nonexistent beds. The wall alcoves where the beds' heads should be are banked by switches marked EXAMINATION LIGHT and EMERGENCY. Next to the window, which looks out on the steel and glass face of a new research building called the New Research Building, is the door to a little bathroom whose sink has foot pedals for faucets. In front of the window are Stickgold's desk, a few books, and two file cabinets, the only items in the room that signal its new life as an office. On top of the file cabinets are three enormous blue binders, one marked "Cognition," one marked "fMRI," and one marked "Tetris." Next to them is an albino hamster. It is wearing sunglasses and a bright yellow disco shirt and has blond hair that looks as if it were treated with Jheri Kurl. Sometimes the hamster sings "Play That Funky Music White Boy."

Beyond Stickgold's office is a conference room known as the solarium, where he took me the day we first met. That day, as we sat before a bank of windows with a sweeping view of Boston, he told me how he'd come to study sleep. A self-described aging hippie with gray hair brushed straight back from his forehead;* fair, freckled skin; and teeth crowded into a pursed, almost rosebud mouth, Stickgold said, "For whatever reason, when I was in sixth grade I decided I was going to be a scientist. No clue why. I just have that fact." And even though as a boy growing up in Chicago he was interested in (or perhaps obsessed with) sleep—to the extent that he would lie awake wondering what would happen after he was asleep, tortured with the idea that he'd be oblivious to whatever it was—he never thought of going into sleep research, a field still in its infancy when he went to college.

Instead, when he was a freshman in high school, six years after Francis Crick and James Watson described DNA's structure, Stickgold

---

* It is carefully cut and styled, every six weeks, by a middle-aged man named Clinton, whom I visited with Stickgold the second day I spent with him. Clinton has a fluffy white and hyperexcitable dog named Max, cites Mark Twain ("he never let his schooling interfere with his education") and quotes Milton ("Quips and Cranks, and wanton Wiles / Nods, and Becks, and Wreath'd Smiles") as he clips, and told us that his haircuts are based on the first axiom in plane geometry (which says that the shortest distance between two points is a straight line).

told me, "I read an article in *Scientific American* where they were try-ing to decide whether the genetic code was a triplet code or a quadru-plet code." We now know it is a triplet code, with each triad of nucleic acids in a gene representing one amino acid to be added to a protein. At the time, however, it was still an open question, with some re-searchers theorizing that evolution might have selected for a more rigid quadruplet code, which would obviate certain mutations allowed by the triplet code. "So I read that article," Stickgold said, "and I actu-ally understood it. And I decided that I was going to be a biochemist. Freshman year in high school. And being sort of the ultimate geeky nerd, I went on to become a biochemist."

His high school nerdiness, which led him to take enough ad-vanced science classes that he entered college at Harvard as a sopho-more, turned out to have been lucky. The year he finished there was the last during the Vietnam War in which he could get a draft defer-ment by enrolling in graduate school. "Everybody else who entered with me," he said, "had to either start doing volunteer work or get braces on their teeth," because conditions requiring regular medical attention brought exemption from the draft. So without resorting to orthodontia, Stickgold avoided the war by becoming a PhD candi-date at the University of Wisconsin at Madison, where he studied DNA replication in bacteria.

Despite his strict adherence to the fifteen-year plan he'd laid out for himself as a teenager, there were a couple of hints along the way that Stickgold might be more interested in humans than in bacteria. While still in high school, he began reading Russell and Whitehead's *Principia Mathematica* for a math project. "The introduction is all I got through, one hundred pages of the introduction," he told me, but said he remembers deciding then to come up with a mathematical equation explaining women, a goal he said was indicative "of both my absolute bafflement at the other sex and my belief that it would be ul-timately reducible."

Stickgold—who at the time we met had recently married his third wife and was, at fifty-eight, about to become a father for the fourth time—ultimately abandoned hope of finding such an equation, but his interest in the human mind remained. He remembers a graduate student at the lab where he worked during high school telling him that all the bacterial research they were doing was unimportant and that his true dream was to study the mind, but that science had yet to develop the right tools to do so. Remembering his friend's comment, Stickgold later took a couple of undergraduate psychology courses at Harvard but came to the same conclusion himself and continued on his bacterial path.

Yet Stickgold audited a neurobiology course even while working on his PhD, and both of his postdoctoral jobs—first in a lab where he studied nerve growth factor,* and then in a neurophysiologist's lab back at Harvard—showed a leaning toward the brain. While in Cambridge, he attended what must have been a very affecting speech by Woody Guthrie's widow, who visited Harvard while trying to drum up interest in studying neurologic diseases, particularly Huntington's disease, the genetic degenerative condition that killed Guthrie. In one sense, she failed in her mission, at least in Stickgold's case, because he moved even further from the field of neurologic research. But she did make an impact on him. After hearing her speech, he told me, "I just thought that I should do politically relevant scientific research." That decision, along with a couple of other factors that included his courageous but ill-received attempt to work only forty hours a week during his postdoc, explains why he ended up at the University of Massachusetts Medical School—a step down in

---

* NGF is a compound made in our bodies that, as its name implies, makes some nerves grow. It is of great interest to neuroscientists because many nerve cells, specifically those in the brain and spinal cord, don't regenerate under normal circumstances. If they could be made to do so, a treatment might be found for damage to the brain and spinal cord from trauma or disease.

prestige from Harvard and Stanford—studying uterine physiology, which was at the time a step down in prestige from almost anywhere.

"This is back when the gynecologist was the absolute bottom of the medical pecking order because he dealt with women's organs. And what could be more gross and disgusting?" Stickgold said. "It was so Neanderthal and so sexist and so despicable. So I decided I would start doing research—that someone had to start doing good research in that area. Just a little quiet Harvard arrogance, but not much." He spent three years at UMass, "writing grants that didn't get funded and not figuring out how to play the game, and ending up really unhappy and feeling isolated," he said. "And so I just left. I literally just told them I was leaving. I didn't have any other job." Such a move is so utterly unheard of that he might as well have pledged never to set foot in an academic lab again.

After that, Stickgold says he "wandered in the desert for forty years," meaning he worked in educational-software development and then did some computer programming, in which he'd been interested since the days when he'd hoped women would be reducible to an equation, "back when sixty-four K was an IBM mainframe and programming was all done on punch cards." His programming work included freelancing for the investment firm Shearson Lehman Brothers, now Lehman Brothers, until one day, "I sort of had the epiphany that I didn't want to tell my grandchildren that I had made the world a better place for Shearson Lehman. So I decided I had made this terrible mistake and I took a couple of courses at the Harvard extension school—one in epistemology and one from Allan Hobson on waking, sleeping, and dreaming." It was 1989, seven years after Stickgold walked out on his faculty job. He was forty-four.

The year he took the course with Hobson, a psychiatrist and one of the big names in sleep research, Stickgold began to work for him as a twenty-hour-a-week programmer at an annual salary of $7,500. Hobson later took him on full-time as a researcher. Ridiculously low salary notwithstanding, at last Stickgold had found his calling. Before that, he says, "my mind was compartmentalized—on one level I was doing cellular neurophys and going on to do uterine physiology, and on another level it was sort of building. You know, it's sort of like adolescent boys who think they hate this girl, and you can just watch it as an adult and say, 'This is love'... I was starting to fall in love with this area that I had been quietly falling in love with since high school."

SLEEP IS ONE of the great unsolved mysteries facing those who, like Stickgold, find themselves fascinated by the human mind. As baffling a problem as consciousness is, once we have accepted that we are conscious, why should we need to lie down and become unconscious for hours at a time every night? Our other daily needs and drives are easier to explain: we have to take in fuel and water to replace what we lose as we burn energy, we have to take shelter to keep our bodies from being destroyed by the elements, we have to have sex to ensure survival of the species. One might question why we are designed to use the kinds of fuel we do, or why we aren't impervious to the elements, or why we aren't individually immortal, but given the way our bodies are made and the way inheritance happens and that we do die, it's pretty clear why we need food, water, shelter, and sex, and why it's hardwired into our bodies to seek those things out.

But there is no obvious reason why we couldn't just keep running, taking in fuel and sheltering from storms and re-creating, without shutting down each night. If we were like cars in the Daytona 500, dependent on outside manipulation to repair the damage caused by a day of living, the immobility sleep forces on us would make sense. But biologically speaking, we carry our pit crew around with us, healing wounds and regrowing hair, skin, and blood from within. There's no intuitive reason to think our immune system or our bodies' regeneration and repair mechanisms need us to hold still while they work. And yet it turns out that forgoing sleep messes with our ride-along maintenance team. Research has shown that people who get less sleep have lowered immune defenses. In addition, some hormones (growth hormone, for instance) are produced only, or in greatest amounts, when we're asleep. But are those processes the reason we sleep, or have they simply evolved to take advantage of the fact that we do?

Most likely the latter, Stickgold thinks, because even if your immune and endocrine systems needed you to lie still for them to work, sleep could simply be a period of forced physical rest. Why don't we just collapse in paralysis each night, our minds remaining alert?

That's not how it works, though. We all spend between a quarter and a third of our lives sleeping, and sleep requires unconsciousness. Our sensory perception shuts off—or somewhere along the line between detection and awareness a switch is flipped and the connection is lost—and we can't *do* anything with our minds, can't plan experiments or run through math problems, can't write sonnets or symphonies or devise political strategies or figure out what we'll make the kids for lunch tomorrow. Science is still at a loss to explain why we should need to do something so radical and seemingly antithetical to survival as sleep, which renders us incapable of gathering food or detecting approaching predators or planning our next move for hours at a time each and every day.

Or why$_f$ we should. Perhaps influenced by his early exposure to *Principia Mathematica* (and certainly influenced by Aristotle, who in his *Physics* discusses the "four causes" that can be provided as answers to the question of why something happens), Stickgold divides the reasons things happen into reasons$_c$ and reasons$_f$. In his notation, the c in *reasons$_c$* stands for "causal" and denotes the mechanistic reasons things happen, while the f in *reasons$_f$* stands for "final" and refers to bigger-picture reasons.* According to his schema, the question of why$_c$ we

---

* Aristotle's four causes were "material," "formal," "efficient," and "final" and referred to the material of which something is made, the plans on which something is made, the method and tools with which something is made, and the final purpose or reason for which something is made. So for instance the material cause of a cake would be flour, eggs, sugar, chocolate, butter, and baking powder; the formal cause of the cake would

sleep can be answered by detailing the physical processes that lead to sleep; the question of why$_f$ we sleep asks why sleep evolved, what it is that makes us need sleep.

The answer to why$_c$ we sleep has been figured out to some extent. As that answer began to be elucidated, it became clear that sleep isn't simply a shutting down of active brain processes, as many had assumed. Normally, when you're awake, neurons in the hypothalamus, which is about the size of the head of a toothbrush and located just above the pituitary gland, are steadily firing and releasing histamine. The histamine released by the hypothalamus (in particular by a part of the hypothalamus called the tuberomamillary nucleus) keeps you awake. When the hypothalamus stops releasing histamine, you feel drowsy and fall asleep.

In the rest of your body, histamine is released by immune cells in inflammatory reactions such as those caused by allergies, which is why you take an antihistamine when you have hay fever. Histamine's role in keeping us awake was not known when the first antihistamines were developed to treat allergies, but anyone who's ever taken Benadryl has experienced the crushing drowsiness it causes when it crosses the blood-brain barrier and blocks the histamine receptors in the brain. That side effect has since been exploited by the pharmaceutical companies in the repackaging of diphenhydramine hydrochloride, the active ingredient in Benadryl, as a sleep aid. (Sominex, for example, is diphenhydramine hydrochloride. The dosage is exactly the same as that in Benadryl.)

---

be the recipe; the efficient cause would be the baker and her KitchenAid; and the final cause would be "for dessert" or "because it tastes good" or "so I can make money selling it" or "because society has told me that women are cake bakers and therefore I ought to be the one to make the cake for my son's birthday party." Or whatever. In Stickgold's division, the "final reason" is the same as Aristotle's "final cause," and Stickgold's "causal why" could probably be considered an amalgam of Aristotle's other three causes.

So what makes the tuberomammilary nucleus of the hypothalamus stop releasing histamine when we go to sleep? The answer, according to Stickgold—who has diagnosed himself with a light case of attention-deficit/hyperactivity disorder and claims he never reads the scientific literature—is "it's complicated." But he broke it down into an ADHD-size chunk: Your circadian clock, which regulates your body's daily cycles, is kept by another part of the hypothalamus called the suprachiasmatic nucleus. It sits just above the optic chiasm and keeps track of how much light you're exposed to by sampling the information streaming through your optic nerves. Based on that data, it sends out signals to the rest of the brain. It's probably the suprachiasmatic nucleus that tells your tuberomammilary nucleus to make you feel sleepy on midwinter afternoons when it begins to get dark just a couple of hours after lunch, and to wake you up at five thirty on June mornings when it's light at that hour.*

Other areas in the brain influence the hypothalamus and cortex to make you fall asleep or keep you awake—most notably a part of the brain stem called the ascending reticular activating system. Finally, there is your conscious mind. If your conscious mind is active and worrying about whether you'll get into medical school or find true love or give a good speech to your company's stockholders, or if it's excitedly anticipating your first day of school or your third date or your IPO, it's hard to fall asleep. We don't know a causal reason for that one, how your thoughts keep your hypothalamus actively releasing histamine.

---

* And what about people blinded by cataracts, so that no (or very little) light makes it to the retina to send signals down the optic nerve? The neurons in the suprachiasmatic nucleus actually have a default twenty-five-hour clock built in, so in the absence of light, they just send out their messages based on that. Which probably would make blind people tend to get out of whack with the rest of the world's timing, were it not for the other things by which we live our lives—alarm clocks, families—that have more influence on us than a little skew in our circadian rhythms.

Once you are asleep, though, the neurons just above the hypothalamus, in the thalamus, start a slow, rhythmic firing. The thalamus is the central switching station in the brain that most sensory information has to pass through before we become conscious of it, and the firing of those thalamic neurons apparently blocks that sensory information, making us deaf to most sounds, blind even to the phosphenes we see when we're awake with our eyes closed, and unable to feel the bed beneath us. But why?

Stickgold's research aim is to find out what happens during sleep, from which he hopes to learn why it is so vital to our existence. To do that, he uses fMRI ("nude photos, we call them"), polysomnographs (a kind of physiologic monitoring system), and video games. When I spent the night hooked up to the computer in Stickgold's lab, I was serving as a control in one of his experiments. The job had required me to play four hours of the arcade game Alpine Racer during the previous day. Consisting of a video screen, a pair of poles, and two slats mounted on a platform, the game requires a player to manipulate the slats with her feet, guiding a digital alter ego through the turns necessary to avoid flags, cliff faces, and other animated skiers. Stickgold believes that by asking his subjects to play the game, he will be able to control their dreams.

He has been gathering evidence to support that theory since his first foray into the field of video-games-as-research-tools. That experiment involved an old standby of the gamishly inclined intelligentsia, the computer game that—before the days of online megagames and guts-and-graphics fests like Carmageddon (billed on at least one Web site as "Bloody Combat Apocalyptic Auto Deathracing")—was so popular it was once rumored to be part of a plot by the Soviet Union to take over the world: Tetris. One day while I was visiting him, I accompanied Stickgold to a seminar at one of Harvard's houses, where he spoke in a dark wood-paneled room to a group of earnest undergrads eating sweet-and-sour tofu off orange cafeteria trays. "I love talking about this," he told them as he described the phenomenon that led him to use Tetris to study dreaming, "because it's been staring us in the face for twenty-five years."

In 1985, Alexey Pazhitnov, Dmitri Pavlovski, and Vadim Gerasimov developed a game that, as many will recall, involves the efficient packing of seven different shapes. The shapes, made up of varying arrangements of unit squares, fall from the top of a video screen. Using computer keys to rotate the shapes as they fall, you try to stack the shapes with no spaces between them. If you fail to do this, the shapes pile up to the top of the screen, at which point you lose the game. If you are successful, solid lines made from the shapes will disappear, and the new pieces will fall faster, requiring ever speedier judgment and ever more dexterous finger movements. The game is absurdly addictive, and many of us who played it obsessively remember disturbing visions of ghostly Tetris pieces falling down the inside of our eyelids as we tried to sleep the first few nights we'd played the game.

It was a common phenomenon—Stickgold claims that when he lectures at MIT, 80 percent of his audience will recall experiencing it—but it seems to have slid under the scientific radar. Until one day years ago when Stickgold went hiking. He left early in the morning and was back home by two or three in the afternoon, after a particularly tough climb. When he went to bed that night, though, he lay down in bed, closed his eyes, and suddenly felt like he was back on the mountain. He could actually feel the rock under his fingers, he told me—a hallucination so real it startled him awake. He let himself doze off, and it happened again. He tried to think of something else, but soon found himself once more reexperiencing his hike. Then he fell asleep.

When he woke a couple of hours later, Stickgold was curious whether the images and sensations of being back on the mountain would reappear as he tried to fall asleep again. They didn't, which he found strange. "After all," he said, "I had first gone to bed eight hours after getting home, at least ten hours since climbing that segment of trail, and now it was only two hours later. But they were gone. I even tried to imagine myself back there again, but the strength of the illusion was gone. Something had changed in those two hours."

Stickgold later had similar experiences, once after taking a boat trip and running some difficult rapids, and again after skiing. Although scientists had never studied the phenomenon, he found he was not the first person to notice it. In one of his papers on the topic, he quotes a passage from Robert Frost's 1914 poem "After Apple-Picking":

> But I was well
> Upon my way to sleep before it fell,
> And I could tell
> What form my dreaming was about to take.
> Magnified apples appear and disappear,
> Stem end and blossom end,
> And every fleck of russet showing clear.
> My instep arch not only keeps the ache,
> It keeps the pressure of a ladder-round.
> I feel the ladder sway as the boughs bend.
> And I keep hearing from the cellar bin
> The rumbling sound
> Of load on load of apples coming in.

He wanted to study the strange sleep-onset imagery, but, he told me, "every time I thought of putting in an application to our human-studies review board to take novices downhill skiing or white-water rafting, I just laughed." Then, at a lab meeting, he complained about not having found a safe way to elicit the phenomenon, and one of his students remembered having such an experience with Tetris.

At her suggestion, Stickgold recruited two groups of undergraduates: "novices," who had never played Tetris before, and "experts," who had played the game extensively but not recently. He also gathered a handful of subjects with amnesia similar to HM's,* who, as far as anyone knew, had no experience with the game. Stickgold asked all participants to play seven hours of Tetris over three days: an initial session of two hours followed by an hour that same evening, and then an hour in the morning and another in the evening for the next two days.

At night participants slept wearing a contraption called the Nightcap. Developed by Stickgold and his collaborators, the Nightcap provides a simple way of determining if subjects are asleep. It consists of a motion detector and an eyelid-movement sensor, both linked to a computer. Those sensors are stitched into a bandanna (usually—when the Nightcap was used by astronauts on the Mir space station, the sensors were attached to a tennis headband). When the sensors relay that the subject is lying completely still, with eyelids quiescent, the computer judges her to be sleeping.

As they lay in bed wearing the Nightcap, subjects in Stickgold's study were periodically prompted by the computer to record what was going through their minds. At varying intervals, several times before they fell asleep and then a few times afterward, the computer asked them to dictate descriptions of their thoughts, images, and feelings into a microcassette recorder.

The amnesics, of course, had to be led to the computer each day for their Tetris sessions and reinstructed in the rules of the game. This task was taken on by an extremely patient undergraduate who also sat with the amnesic subjects as they fell asleep, turning on the tape

---

* While the removal of both hippocampuses that HM underwent is no longer done, one of the hippocampuses may be removed to treat intractable epilepsy. If such a patient later has a stroke that causes damage to the other hippocampus, she may end up in the same straits that HM is in. Of course, strokes that damage both hippocampuses can also cause such an amnesia. The subjects in Stickgold's study had likely suffered one of the latter two fates.

recorder at the computer's prompt and asking them to describe what they had been seeing, thinking, and feeling.

By the end of the three days of playing Tetris, the nonamnesic novices were nearly as good as the experts, whereas the amnesics hardly got any better at all. That's somewhat surprising, of course, given what we know about HM and the mirror drawing, but Stickgold decided playing Tetris must somehow require declarative memory.* And in fact, there's some research to show that the hippocampus is necessary for the early stages of learning Tetris, after which it's not used. So it may be that these amnesics, without a serviceable hippocampus, just couldn't get past that first hurdle to the point at which playing the game would rely more on nondeclarative memory. So far, the experiment had shown nothing particularly exciting. That amnesics didn't get any better can be explained, and it doesn't take a Harvard scientist to prove college kids get better at video games with two hours of daily play.

It was the dictated nighttime reports that got Stickgold's work published in the journal *Science*. Half the expert subjects and nine of the twelve healthy novices reported experiencing nighttime Tetris-related imagery. Interestingly, there were more reports on the second night than on the first, and most of the reports were the same: Subjects saw Tetris pieces falling down in front of their faces. They didn't see themselves at a computer, didn't even see a computer; they just saw Tetris pieces. And most of that visual imagery was recorded after the subjects had been deemed by the Nightcap to be asleep. Some of the expert players, who had learned the game with a different version than the bare-bones black-and-white one Stickgold had them

---

* Remember, *declarative* means "explicit" and refers to memories such as what you had for breakfast this morning or who is the president right now, whereas *nondeclarative* means "implicit" or "procedural" and refers to skill memories, such as how to ride a bike or ski.

playing, saw colored Tetris pieces they identified as being from the version of the game they'd first played on.

That Stickgold had found a way to influence people's minds after they fell asleep, and that he seemed able to compel them to recall old Tetris memories, were both mildly surprising. Even more surprising, though, was that three of the five amnesic subjects also reported seeing shapes drifting down in front of their eyes. Their descriptions of those shapes were unmistakably of Tetris pieces. Stickgold's paper on the study includes some of what those subjects—who couldn't even remember the word Tetris—said. "I was just trying to figure out those shapes and how to get them aligned," one of them reported. "Thinking about little squares coming down on a screen and trying to put them in place," said another. A third said, "Images that are turned on their side. I don't know what they are from—I wish I could remember—but they are like blocks."

WHILE STICKGOLD USED the Nightcap in the Tetris experiment to determine when subjects had fallen asleep, a polysomnograph, which is what I wore while sleeping in his lab, provides both more elaborate and more subtle information to researchers about their sleeping subjects. Polysomnographs consist of an electroencephalogram as well as an electromyogram and an electrooculogram. The electromyogram and electrooculogram are readouts from sensors stuck beneath a subject's chin and beside the eye, respectively. The electromyogram records muscle tone, and the electrooculogram tracks the eye's movement.

The many neurons in your brain, both the ones doing your thinking as you read this and the ones acting outside your consciousness, keeping your breathing going and signaling for hormone release and consolidating memories and so on, are doing so by means of the electrical firing that Christof Koch measures in his experiments with epileptic patients' implanted electrodes. But the electroencephalogram, or EEG, part of a polysomnograph records the average of all the neuronal firings in the brain that can be detected at the surface of the scalp. It is created using the readings from electrodes affixed to the subject's scalp with an electrically conductive glue.

It's important to remember that, unlike the microelectrodes Koch uses, an EEG's electrodes measure the net activity of billions of neurons, not any one neuron. As Stickgold says, "You've got about as much chance of figuring out what individual neurons are doing from an EEG as you have standing outside Fenway Park during a Red Sox game, trying to listen to the conversation of the person in section twelve, seat AA forty-seven." What you can pick up, he says, is the neural equivalent of the BoSox fans' response to a home run.

Generally speaking, when you're awake with your eyes open, there are no home runs. An EEG trace from your brain as you're sitting here reading this would look something like this:

Basically, just electrical noise.

Now close your eyes and relax for a moment, trying not to think about anything.

While you had your eyes closed, your brain would have produced an EEG with rhythmic spikes in electrical activity, like this:

For some reason, when you close your eyes, millions of neurons get together and fire synchronously so that they can be picked up with electrodes from outside the skull the way the roar of the crowd after a home run can be picked up by your ears outside a baseball stadium. These waves of synchronous neuronal action are called alpha waves. The phenomenon is generally associated with the lack of input from your eyes to your visual cortex, but no one really understands why it happens.

If when you closed your eyes you started to drift off to sleep, your brain waves would, suprisingly, start to look more like waking, open-eye brain waves than the alpha waves did. In fact, from your brain waves it would be hard to tell if you were asleep or had popped wide awake, with your eyes open. The polysomnograph's muscle-tone sensor allows researchers to differentiate between the two states. If a subject is falling asleep, there will be a drop in her muscle tone; if she came suddenly awake, there would be a little jump in her muscle tone.

Also, as you're falling asleep, your eyes start rolling back and forth, slowly, from side to side. They go from one side to the other and back again with a period of about four seconds. Scientists like Stickgold have agreed—although it's a somewhat arbitrary line they have drawn—that sleep onset occurs when those three criteria have been met: alpha waves disappear, muscle tone drops, and rolling eye movements start. Once those things happen, you're in stage 1 sleep.

Normally, after just a few minutes, you pass from stage 1 to stage 2 sleep. Stage 2 is characterized by typical waveforms known as K complexes, and by sharp series of spikes in the brain's overall electrical activity known as spindles. One feature common to all stages of sleep is that the sleeper is relatively unresponsive to outside stimuli. (Even in stage 1 sleep, during which people often feel awake and are easier to arouse than in the other stages, you can whisper their names quietly and they won't respond.) But K complexes can be elicited by outside stimuli. For instance, Stickgold says that if he had you asleep and hooked up to an EEG, he could stand in the next room and clap, and despite the fact that you wouldn't wake up and wouldn't remember having heard anything—perhaps wouldn't have heard anything, if we take the word *hear* to mean the conscious awareness of an aural stimulus—a K complex would appear on your EEG. Another clap, another K complex would appear.

*There are two K complexes in this trace—they are the tall spikes
and subsequent dips.*

Most K complexes seem not to be caused by outside events, though, and nobody knows what causes them in those cases, or what it means that outside events can cause them.

Stage 2 sleep is also characterized by sleep spindles. "What I find so delightful," Stickgold has written about spindles, "is the precision of their waveform. Remember, we've got an electrode glued to someone's scalp and that electrode is picking up the aggregate activation of a huge fraction of the nerve cells in the brain, and the sum of all this activity, measured more than an inch from most of the cells being recorded, follows this precise shape."

There are always, Stickgold says, six to seven spindles per half second during stage 2 sleep, and almost never any spindles in any other stage of sleep. "Furthermore, the regularity of shape of the overall spindle, both from spindle to spindle and from wave to wave within a spindle, seems exceptional given the variability seen in other brain wave forms."

After stage 2 and the sleep spindles come two more numbered stages. Stages 3 and 4 are the deepest sleep stages, meaning that people are the most difficult to arouse during them. Both stages are characterized by slow, broad, high-amplitude, and regularly repeating waves known as delta waves.

In stages 2 through 4, the slow, unified background waves are attributed, at least in part, to those slow bursts sent out from the thalamus to widely distributed areas of cortex.

About half an hour after you have fallen asleep, you will have moved through stages 1–4 of sleep. Then, like a yo-yo reaching the end of its string, you ascend through the stages again, in reverse order, from 4 to 3 to 2 to 1, although stage 1 sleep, when it's reached from stage 2 rather than from the waking state, is called REM sleep. In REM, your eyes move, as in stage 1, but in REM they dart furiously from left to right and up and down, making the trip from side to side in less than a second. Which is why, of course, REM is called REM, for rapid eye movement. It's also called paradoxical sleep, because although you are asleep, your brain waves, as measured by the EEG, look almost as they would if you were awake: no home runs, just the electrical noise of the activity of millions or billions of individually active neurons.

There is an even greater drop in your muscle tone when you reach REM sleep than there is during the transition from the waking state to stage 1 sleep. In fact, you have essentially no muscle tone at all during REM. Pretty much all mammals have to sleep, as we do, although the number of hours needed varies by species,* and as far as science can tell they all have the paralysis associated with REM sleep. According to Stickgold, even animals like horses that can sleep standing up have to lie down for REM sleep. In normal people, most movement during sleep—grinding teeth, rolling over, and so on—happens during other, non-REM stages. In humans, only a few muscle twitches ever get through the paralysis of REM, most notably those

* Research has shown that brown bats sleep about twenty hours out of each day, while African elephants appear to need only about three hours of sleep per day.

of the muscles that move our eyes. Animals that are less visually oriented, or whose eyes don't move as ours do, don't have rapid eye movements during their analog to REM sleep, but they may have a similar movement that breaks through the paralysis. For instance, rats, who rely on the vibrations from their whiskers to sense the world around them, twitch their whiskers.

The one other physically observable manifestation of REM sleep is that we get erections. Men (and those they sleep with) are familiar with the phenomenon of penile erections arising throughout the night, and men usually awaken in the morning with an erection, since they usually pass through REM sleep on their way to waking up. Women, although they may not know it, also experience this phenomenon, with clitoral swelling accompanying each episode of REM sleep (you cycle up and down through the stages of sleep, hitting REM about once every ninety minutes throughout the night). Nobody knows why($_f$) these erections happen, but then nobody knows the final reason for anything that happens during REM, including the most astonishing phenomenon: dreaming.

As far as scientists can tell, dreams are universally experienced if not universally remembered. Stickgold says that those who protest they never dream are wrong: they just never remember dreaming. If awakened during REM sleep, they'd almost certainly report dreams if asked. Incidentally, during those dreams—unlike their depiction in soap operas, in which dreaming involves thrashing around and calling out for a long-lost twin sister suspected to have been abducted by aliens—our muscles' paralysis renders us completely motionless, but for our eyes.

Babies spend about 50 percent of their sleep time in REM, which, since they sleep most of the day, means they spend about eight hours a day in REM sleep. Normal, healthy, non-sleep-deprived adults ("and therefore *ab*normal," as Stickgold says) usually spend about 20 percent of their sleeping time in REM, or about ninety minutes a day. Your first episode of REM lasts only a couple of minutes, but as you cycle up and down through the stages of sleep, each successive episode grows progressively longer. Contrary to another popular myth that says that dream time doesn't correspond with actual time, Stickgold says we dream "more or less in real time." Those dreams in which you are in your old high school, searching for the room in which your final exam is to be held and marching *forever* through corridor after corridor, probably really do take a long time, at least forty-five minutes or so, which is roughly the length of your REM episodes by the end of your sleeping night.

WHEN I FIRST MET Stickgold, he was an assistant professor of psychiatry at Harvard Medical School and had recently gained his academic independence from Hobson. Most scientists his age would already be full professors—he says he frequently gets calls from people to whom he's just sent his CV, asking for an updated version that includes his current title—but then, most academic scientists his age didn't go wandering in the desert of investment banking in the middle of their careers. His stint away from academia means that Stickgold is still working on developing collaborative relationships. The day after I served as a subject in the Alpine Racer study (in which Stickgold is attempting to elicit tactile experiences at sleep onset), Stickgold and I ate lunch at Beth Israel. We were joined by a young neurologist who was considering working on a study with Stickgold.

As we sat down amid the echoing racket of hundreds of lunchers, Stickgold began recounting an argument he once had with a philosopher. The philosopher had posed a question about the fusiform gyrus, the bit of cortex activated when people see and remember faces. The question, according to Stickgold, was whether the fusiform gyrus could, in theory, be conscious of a face, could *experience* a face, without out the rest of the self's being conscious of that face. If so, he wondered, how could science determine that the fusiform gyrus was having the experience? "That was his big question," Stickgold said over a slice of cafeteria pizza.

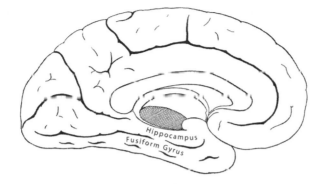

"It's been done," said the young neurologist, who wore a yellow tie printed with blue frogs. "It's been done thirty years ago by Damasio.* The answer is yes. Those agnosics who don't recognize faces have galvanic skin responses to familiar faces but not to unfamiliar faces."

The galvanic skin response is used frequently in cognitive experiments. It is also one component of a lie-detector test. Both uses require electrodes applied to the skin, usually at the fingertips. The skin's ability to conduct electricity increases as the moisture on it increases; even tiny changes in sweat output, undetectable by sight or touch, can be picked up by testing the skin's conductivity. In polygraph tests, an increase in galvanic skin response (along with increases in other physiologic measures such as heart rate and blood pressure) is taken to be a sign of the stress induced by lying. In research, the galvanic skin response is also usually used to detect stress.

An agnosic has intact sensory capacities but has brain damage that makes certain kinds of recognition impossible. The most commonly described agnosias are visual. People with visual object agnosia may not be able to visually recognize an everyday object such as a pen but if allowed to feel the object will have no trouble identifying it. There are agnosias of the other senses as well. Some agnosics are able to recognize an object by sight but not by feel, for instance. The

---

* Antonio Damasio, a neurologist and researcher and the author of *The Feeling of What Happens* and other books on the mind and brain.

subjects in the experiment the neurologist mentioned had prosopagnosia, an inability to recognize faces by sight in someone with otherwise normal vision.

It's uncanny but no longer surprising, given what we are now learning about the multiple unconscious perceptual systems in the brain, that prosopagnosics show some signs of visually "recognizing" faces even while not consciously recognizing them. In Damasio's experiment, four people with face agnosia were shown pictures of faces, some of which they'd seen before, some of which they hadn't. Although all the subjects denied familiarity with any of the faces, their galvanic skin response increased each time they were shown a picture of a face that they had, in fact, seen before.

Stickgold doesn't think the results of that study answer the philosopher's question, though. "The question is," he says, "could one part of the brain be *experiencing* the qualia associated with a face, without the rest of the brain? Or as I asked him, 'Can you be aware of something without being aware of it?' and he said, 'Yes.' And I said, 'Well, that's easy. Either *aware* means two different things that I don't understand, or else the answer is no. The Greeks figured that out, right?"

According to Stickgold, the philosopher then asked whether, if you cut all the connections leading out of the fusiform gyrus to the rest of the brain, leaving all the incoming connections intact (a thought experiment impossible in practice), the fusiform gyrus could have the experience of a face without the owner of the fusiform gyrus experiencing sight of the face.

"Wittgenstein," the neurologist said now, "argued that, at the fundamental level, you and I could never completely agree on the definition of any single word—especially a word like *consciousness*. And if you can't, if it's absolutely irreducible and it can never be proven that you and I mean the same thing when we mean 'consciousness' or 'awareness,' then it's futile to try to develop a whole system around something that at its fundament is not sound."

"You don't mean that we can't agree," said Stickgold. "It's that we can't agree and actually know that. We could agree. We could both agree that this is yellow." He pointed to the background on the neurologist's tie.

"Correct. But I would never know that my perception of yellow is your perception of yellow. And usually for day-to-day function it's not a major impediment. But when you get into a very detailed discussion on what you mean by *awareness* and *consciousness* and *subconsciousness,* that's all that's left." This type of debate, the neurologist said, highlighted the reason he is wary of researching consciousness. "At the end of the day you're gonna sound like a bunch of college sophomores late at night, sleep deprived, talking about 'do I mean what you mean when I perceive what you perceive.'"

Stickgold agreed, mentioning a colleague with whom he'd gotten into an argument when "he said that our Coke machine might have a low level of consciousness because it receives input and then responds to a perceived need and gives people what they want."

"Let me ask you a question," the neurologist said. "If you've got a Coke machine in Wisconsin, sitting in front of a gas station, and it's got a little cooler in it to keep the Cokes nice and cold in the summertime—when it gets to minus thirty, does it have a little heater in there to prevent the suckers from freezing?"

As STICKGOLD'S COLLEAGUE pointed out, one of the many difficulties arising as a result of new discoveries in cognitive neuroscience is that words whose meanings have long been clear are now hazy. When you talk about memory today, what are you talking about? Conscious memories? If so, what name should we give to our unconscious memories, which are proving to be more vast and important than previously thought? And once you have that sorted out, where do you draw the line between conscious and unconscious? The amnesics in Stickgold's Tetris experiment were certainly conscious of the imagery they perceived as they fell asleep, but not of what to associate it with.

Stickgold told me he once did a simple study in which he gave his students a questionnaire and asked them to fill it out when they awoke after a dream. He found, among other things, that 16 percent of the people who popped up in his students' dreams were unknown to the students; they didn't recognize them at all. Could those people be real — people the dreamers had met but forgotten? And if so, what does *forgotten* mean if you can retain, somewhere in your brain, the ability to call up the image of the forgotten person, just as the amnesics stored mental images of Tetris pieces without knowing what they were?

When Stickgold brought up the philosopher's question about the fusiform gyrus, it was to make fun; he doesn't think it's a useful question. But now that we have fMRI data suggesting that your brain may be "smelling" odors without *your* smelling them, and given that a subject's brain might be "hearing" Stickgold clap his hands in the next room without the subject's hearing the sound herself — and that your own brain, like HM's and the Tetris amnesics', may be remembering things you don't — what will we do about the verbs we've been tossing around so casually, as if your brain's detecting something and your detecting it were the same thing? Will we have to take a page from Stickgold's book and talk about whether we hear$_s$ or hear$_b$ things, where *s* stands for "self" and *b* stands for "brain"? Was the philosopher with whom Stickgold argued right to be wondering if your fusiform gyrus, cut off from sending messages to the rest of your brain, might have its own experience of your grandmother's face even while you don't? If one of Koch's subjects' neurons — say, one that fires when its owner is shown a picture of Jennifer Aniston — was removed from the subject's brain, kept alive in a petri dish and stimulated with a micro-electrode, would it have the experience of those bright eyes and that sassy smile?

The confusion is everywhere, as we begin to discover that what we thought were unified ideas can actually be broken down into discrete pieces. One of the words coming under new scrutiny is written in script made of glass tubing and leaned up against the window behind Stickgold's desk: "dream."

"In the final submission," of the Tetris grant proposal, Stickgold told me, "I took the word 'dreaming' out of the proposal entirely, because one of the reviewers said I wasn't studying dreaming; I was studying hypnagogic imagery, not dreaming." According to that reviewer, he said, "dreams are narratives—with people in them, and things happening, and emotions that are relevant to emotional experiences in their everyday life." Under which characterization Stickgold's subjects' Tetris imagery didn't qualify.

Stickgold disagrees with such a strict definition. Although he admits he's not sure what dreaming is, either, he says he's pretty sure it's not so cut-and-dried. Stickgold was part of a consensus group organized by the Associated Professional Sleep Societies and charged with arriving at a definition of the word *dream*. At the group's final meeting, he said, "The conclusion was that we are nowhere close to having a consensus definition of dreaming, that there are some very respected people that say dreaming should not be limited to the time when you're asleep, that daydreams—if they are significantly separate from where you are and what you're doing—are as much dreams as anything else. And there are other people who say if it's not in REM sleep, it's not real dreaming. And there are some people who say if it doesn't have certain features, it isn't real dreaming." Which, he pointed out, raises the question of what to call all the phenomena not falling under the umbrella of dreaming. And so, he said, "in the final grant application that got approved, I said, 'OK, I won't study dreaming. I'll study sleep-onset mentation.'" Nevertheless, he thinks we can probably consider the strange, hallucinatory images experienced by subjects in his Tetris experiments to be dreams. If true, of course, that would mean he's found a revolutionary way to control dream content and so explore the question of how our waking life influences our dreaming life (and perhaps vice versa).

The fact that no one can agree on the definition of dreaming reflects the fact that, as with the rest of the phenomena associated with sleep, no one knows why we do it. But Stickgold, along with other researchers, is beginning to collect evidence to support the idea that one of sleep's purposes may be to help us learn. An experiment he did in 2002 serves as a good example. For the study, he and his collaborators asked a group of right-handed college-age subjects to practice a task either at ten in the morning or at ten in the evening. Their assignment was to type the sequence 4-1-3-2-4 as fast as they could, as many times as they could, for thirty seconds. Then they were asked to do the same thing for eleven more thirty-second intervals, with thirty-second rests between the intervals. The catch was, they were to do all the typing with their left hands. Naturally, over the course of this training period, all subjects, whether trained in the morning or the evening, improved at the task. The subjects were scored based on how many correct sequences they could produce in their allotted thirty seconds. Over the entire twelve minutes of training, they got about 60 percent better at the task.

Stickgold's team then sent each group away for twelve hours, testing them again at the end of that time. When the morning-trained group was tested twelve hours later, at 10:00 p.m., they were a tiny bit—about 2 percent—better than when they had finished training that morning. The subjects who'd been trained at 10:00 p.m. were brought back for the second testing at 10:00 a.m. the following morning, after a night's sleep. Without any further training, without any more time between training and testing than the waking group had, those subjects showed an average improvement of 20 percent. Stickgold's group later tested the morning-trained subjects again, without any further training but after they had gotten a night's sleep. On that testing, they also showed an improvement of about 20 percent.

It turned out the subjects' improvement seemed to be correlated with the amount of stage 2 sleep the subjects got, but why that should be is still unclear. Stickgold theorizes the spindles seen in stage 2 sleep may have something to do with such motor learning, but he'd be the first to admit that's just a pet theory borne of his love for sleep spindles. No one knows if he's right, and even if he were, the next question would be why we need the activity producing the spindles to learn motor skills. To add to the confusion, there are other studies correlating such skill learning with REM sleep or stage 3 and 4 sleep, rather than with stage 2 sleep. Regardless of when it occurs, however, it's clear *something* is happening during sleep that allows us—without further practice—to improve at skills requiring non-declarative memory. Other studies Stickgold conducted have shown that, even without additional training, subjects continue to get better and better at a task across several nights of sleep. But his studies also show that if subjects are not allowed further practice, those who miss that first night of sleep after training are never able to catch up with those who do get a night's sleep.

Scientists have long surmised that one of the reasons$_f$ we sleep, and possibly one of the reasons$_f$ we dream, is to consolidate our memories. When scientists began talking about sleep and memory consolidation, they usually assumed—probably because dreaming is so richly experiential and, as Stickgold's reviewer pointed out, is usually narrative—that sleep had something to do with laying down and preserving declarative memories, memories of events. No one has been able to convincingly demonstrate such an association, however. But studies such as Stickgold's show that, at least in the short term, sleep is vital for laying down nondeclarative memories. The fact that the amnesics, who had no idea where the shapes came from, reported Tetris images as they fell asleep makes it likely that whatever memory system those images arise from, it isn't declarative memory. And the 4-1-3-2-4 task at which Stickgold's subjects improved after sleep is purely nondeclarative. So Stickgold has taken to recommending that the first night after you learn to ski or surf or knit or type or ride a bicycle or play the violin, you should get a good night's sleep. And presumably, as you keep practicing those skills, one of the easiest ways to speed up your improvement at your newly acquired skill is to make sure you get enough sleep.*

STICKGOLD LIKES TO SAY that he studies consciousness by studying unconsciousness, and the morning I arrived at his office door after spending the night in his sleep lab, he had promised me he'd give me his theory of consciousness. To do so, he took me down the hall to the solarium again, where we sat down. Once we were settled, he told me that on the subject of consciousness, "the most fundamental place I come down is abject ignorance. Which is where we should all be."

Neither that attitude nor the fact that the purpose of sleep and dreaming remains mysterious means Stickgold doesn't have his own theory of how the two contribute to the fancy consciousness that mammals (maybe, to some extent) and humans (certainly) enjoy. If true, his theory would also help explain why it is that in order to have such a consciousness within the constraints provided by the size and workings of our brains, we have to sleep.

Remember Terry Dibert, who was found wandering along the highway and, before the removal of the cyst blocking communication between his hippocampus and the rest of his brain, was unable to recall declarative memories from the previous decade or so of his life. We know that over some period of time — years, apparently — declar-

---

* The first thing that came to my mind when I heard about these data was Glick's surgical resident, Mike Song, who was learning how to do the manipulations required to cut open people's heads and remove parts of their brains. Medical training is set up so that he gets less sleep, far less sleep, than the rest of us, spending at least eighty hours a week on duty. Many doctors, even many residents, argue that without the punishing hours, medicine can't be taught properly. They say it's vital for doctors in training to see the number and variety of cases that such a system allows. Some say that the horrible deprivations residents experience — of sleep, of healthy food, of exercise, of social interaction — are also necessary so that they are able to practice under any conditions. It will take more research like Stickgold's to discover whether these arguments hold water.

ative memories are transferred from the hippocampus to the cortex (or at least access to them is made hippocampus-independent). This lengthy transfer is the reason both HM and Dibert retained memories from some time before their cortices were separated from their hippocampuses but not from immediately before.

Whether the hippocampus acts to store the entirety of the memories during the time in which it is crucial for retrieving them or instead acts as a kind of index, storing links to the cortical areas necessary for the memory, is unclear. (In that case, presumably the cortical areas necessary for the memory eventually become associated strongly enough that they don't need the hippocampus to provide a link between them.) But what seems clear is that some kind of active process must be involved in making the declarative memories independent of the hippocampus, and that once they are, the hippocampus will eventually need to be cleaned out, either of memories or of links to memories, in order to make room for new memories or links to memories.

Another thing we know happens over time is that declarative memories are stripped of all but essential detail—or at least become much less detailed than they originally were. So although today you may remember your first day of high school, that you met Mike then, and that your first class was English, you don't remember what you wore or what you ate for breakfast that day, as you probably did a week later. At the same time, your memory of that day has changed and been associated with other memories acquired since then—all the days you spent in your high school afterward, the fact that Mike later became a curator at the Louvre, your high school reunion, and so on.

Stickgold points out that such a system allows more efficient use of the brain's storage capacity but that for it to work, the brain would logically need to play around with the neurons underlying those memories. That manipulation would likely require the firing of some of those neurons, which, Stickgold feels, would naturally result in a conscious experience. He also argues that we can't very well be throwing new data at the brain as it tries to process the old data of memories.

He believes that sleep, with its enforced isolation from sensory input, is a perfect time for the culling, testing, and transferring of declarative memories and probably evolved for that reason, although he allows that it's kind of silly to talk about sleep serving any one particular purpose. "To talk about the function of sleep is a mistake in the same way as talking about the function of your tongue is," he said. "If you heard two tongue researchers having an argument and one says the tongue is used for tasting food and the other says, 'Nonsense, it's used for articulating speech,' you'd think that they were basically daft, right?"

So while sleep is by now as integrated as our tongues with our body's multiple functions and is advantageous to multiple physiologic processes, he thinks at least three of those processes are mental. First, these include the organization and tweaking of newly acquired nondeclarative memories so that they serve us better the next time we access them, even if we don't receive further training. Second, he theorizes that declarative memories are strengthened, refined, and integrated with one another as we sleep, leading to those memories' future independence from the hippocampus. Finally, he thinks that during sleep, the neocortex and hippocampus compare notes, allowing the hippocampus to erase declarative memories (or links to them) that have been sufficiently cemented into the neocortex.

Because it seems clear to him that fiddling with these memories must involve fiddling with some of the neurons we use for (or whose activity is) consciousness, Stickgold says, "I have now taken to describe dreaming as the phenomenology that unavoidably arises when the neural networks and neural systems necessary for memory processing happen to include a sufficient portion of those which underlie consciousness." It is this capacity to shut our minds down and cull, distill, integrate, and reorganize our memories that Stickgold believes allows our three-pound brains to demonstrate computational and storage capacities that far outstrip the abilities of the largest and most complex computers.

INTERLUDE: Adolescence

Conception	6 weeks	10 weeks	30 weeks	6 years	Adolescence	Adulthood	Old Age	Death

Birth

It used to be thought that after myelination was completed in childhood, our brains' physical development was essentially finished. In 1979, however, the pediatric neurologist Dr. Peter Huttenlocher changed that impression with one small study. For the study, he obtained tiny pieces of the brains of twenty-one neurologically healthy people who had died at ages ranging from newborn to ninety years old. The pieces were taken from the middle frontal gyrus of each brain, and Huttenlocher used an electron microscope to count the synapses in each piece of cortex. His original goal was simply to learn the normal number of synapses in healthy brains of various ages so that he could later compare those values with the number of synapses in abnormal brains. As he had expected, the number of synapses in most of the pieces of brain were about the same. Each sample from subjects between sixteen and seventy-two years old had between 8.9 billion and 12.5 billion synapses per cubic millimeter of cortex. Newborn babies also had numbers of synapses within that range. But Huttenlocher found that the number of synapses increased dramatically after birth. When you were born, you had maybe 10 billion synapses per cubic millimeter of cortex, with more forming every minute. By one year old, you had something on the order of 16.5 billion synapses per cubic millimeter, or about 30 percent more than you have now. After your first birthday, however, the growth of new synapses leveled off. Then sometime between the ages of one and seven, you started to lose synapses. By the time you hit your mid- to late teens, you're back down to the number of synapses you were born with, the number you'll keep—with a possible slight decline in old age—until your death.

That such a dramatic pruning of synapses happens so late in our development was surprising at the time Huttenlocher noted it, although there had been some evidence in animals for a smaller-scale synaptic pruning close to maturity. A few years after he published his results, the psychiatrist and sleep researcher Dr. Irwin Feinberg put forward an entirely new idea based on them. Feinberg was interested in schizophrenia, which frequently emerges during adolescence, and often in children who had until that point appeared entirely normal.

Schizophrenia is a psychotic disorder characterized by hallucinations (such as hearing voices), delusions (for example, that others can read your thoughts), and severe mental disorganization. It remains a mystery how schizophrenia can arise in a brain that has been functioning normally for years. Feinberg suggested that the change might be a consequence of the synaptic pruning Huttenlocher had discovered, and that the dramatically aberrant consciousness of schizophrenia might be caused by a derangement of the pruning process, where either too many, too few, or the wrong synapses were destroyed.

His theory is unproven, and there are many others, most focusing on the role of the neurotransmitter dopamine, whose effects are blocked by the drugs successful in treating schizophrenia. But in 1998, two Yale psychiatrists conducted an experiment that may support Feinberg's theory. They designed a computer simulation of one aspect of cognition: the perception of speech. Their model consisted of 148 interconnected "neural elements." The computer was programmed with strings of symbols representing words. The system could recognize each "word" even if the full string of symbols wasn't given. Thus inputs could be "heard" by the computer even when incomplete, just as we hear human speech even when background noise or a bad cell-phone connection garbles it.

The Yale scientists then simulated synaptic pruning by severing some of the interconnections between processing elements. Up to a point, despite the loss of connections, the computer could still "hear" the input words. After a certain number of "synapses" had been destroyed, however, the computer not only began incorrectly recognizing words, but it also began to "hear" words without any input. The authors of the study suggested such "auditory hallucinations" by the computer might be analogous to the auditory hallucinations present in schizophrenia.

Around the same time that Feinberg put forward his synaptic-pruning hypothesis, he and other researchers discovered additional changes in our brains during adolescence. They found that the amount of time spent in stage 4, one of the deep stages of sleep, decreases by about 50 percent in adolescents compared to values in younger children. The brain's overall metabolic rate also seems to slow down as we reach our teens, so that by the time we hit our twenties, our brains use only about 70 percent of the oxygen they did at age ten. There are also changes in some measurements of brain electrical activity, showing that certain neural responses speed up during late childhood and early adolescence. Finally, in childhood it's easy to learn to speak a new language or play soccer and—as Roberta Glick pointed out—it's possible to bounce back from even drastic brain injuries with full function. Once we hit adolescence, though, it's much harder for an English speaker to learn Spanish or for a novice to become truly good at tennis, and the brain seems to lose some of its ability to overcome damage. Whether our brains lose this childhood plasticity because of synaptic pruning or some other yet-to-be-discovered developmental event remains to be seen.

Oh, shit. I don't want to go there.

—BOB STICKGOLD

5 | Multiple Minds

A FRIEND DROPPED ME OFF. She told me later that as she watched me carrying my purse and notebook up the twisting driveway through the woods obscuring the house I was headed for, she'd wondered if she was doing the right thing in letting me go alone. She wasn't the only one worried: my boyfriend had made me promise the first thing I'd do on arriving would be to note all the house's exits, making sure I had an escape route once inside.

So much concern, when I was simply planning to spend an afternoon in the Hamptons with Judy Castelli, a middle-aged artist and former nightclub singer. Castelli, however, has dissociative identity disorder, formerly known as multiple personality disorder. In addition to sharing the general stigma surrounding all mental illness even in the Prozac era, DID is seen as a kind of shady, culty, "probably not real but I don't really want to think about it anyway" topic fit only for made-for-TV movies and last-minute Hollywood plot twists. At their most apprehensive—especially when faced with the idea of being alone in a room with a DID sufferer—people tend to remember tales of gruesome crimes committed by "dark" personalities or alter egos. That such tales often originated in those same Hollywood plots doesn't mitigate the fear surrounding the illness. Say "multiple personality," and people think of Dr. Jekyll and the terrible Mr. Hyde or imagine inchoate screams and shattering glass set in that eerie, well-lit half dark that exists only to be captured on celluloid.

But when Castelli, a strawberry blond wearing a pink jersey top and striped pedal pushers, came out to meet me holding a coffee mug and accompanied by Dolly, a little multicolored terrier with a bandy-legged trot, the whole scene looked about as scary as a Folgers commercial. In fact, although she shook my hand heartily and asked me inside, Castelli looked a bit wary of me.

The living room into which Castelli led me is filled with sculptures and paintings — on the walls, on the windowsills, and on top of the television. We settled ourselves on a white vinyl sectional behind a rattan and glass coffee table. So far the scariest thing about Castelli was Dolly, who obediently lay down between us when instructed but erupted into sharp, threatening barks whenever I changed position. "If you could just move a little slower," Castelli said, shushing her. Dolly is a service animal, along the lines of a Seeing Eye dog, and Castelli takes her everywhere, as both a companion and a vocal, if physically unimposing, bodyguard.

Almost immediately after sitting down, Castelli seemed to relax a bit. Still, though, "I'll probably need a lot of prompting," she said. "Everything has to filter through so many of us." I asked her how many, exactly, of her there are. "At one point I knew there were forty-four," she said, "and over the years and through treatment I know that number has dwindled a bit, because people tend to overlap now and blend more and kind of join with others. So are there forty-four exactly? Probably not anymore." I asked her if one of her alter identities in particular goes by the name of Judy. "I have three or four that are the adult Judys that sort of present to the room," she said. And then, as casually as mentioning a change in the weather: "So the person that you met on the road," she said, "is a different person than me." She went on. "I'm more comfortable with this process, this talking-about process. The one on the road was kind of more anxious, more nervous, more 'okaaay, let's see,' you know, and probably wouldn't talk a whole lot."

When I later asked my boyfriend what exactly he'd feared would happen to me while I was visiting Castelli, he replied that he'd envisioned radical and polar shifts, "her being charming one minute, then all of a sudden leaping across the room and bludgeoning you to death." I would have been less surprised had that happened. Truthfully, I hadn't been expecting to meet more than one of Castelli's personalities. As she seemed to be living a fairly functional life, I figured she must not switch among them often. But I'd certainly expected to notice if she did — that the change would be dramatic, and the new personality wouldn't remember what the previous one was doing. But this stealth switching?

The psychologist Dr. Daniel Simons, who studies attention and visual cognition, once performed an experiment using an unwitting subject to demonstrate a phenomenon known as change blindness. In the setup, a man in jeans, boots, a tool belt, and a yellow hard hat stops to ask directions of a woman passerby. Unbeknownst to the woman, the exchange is being filmed from a vantage point high above and behind the "worker's" right shoulder. In the middle of their interaction, two more men in construction gear pass between the two, carrying a door. It's obvious from the camera's vantage point that the original hard-hatted man, briefly screened from the woman's view, switches places with one of the men carrying the door. Once the men with the door move out of the way, the replacement construction worker continues the original conversation with the woman as if nothing has happened. Incredibly, the woman does as well. An entirely different person is now before her, receiving the directions for which she'd been asked by the first man, and she doesn't realize a trick has been played.* When Castelli told me she'd switched right in front of me, I felt as Simon's subject must have when she was later shown the tape of herself.

In Castelli's case, of course, there was no change in features that could have tipped me off. But was I, as the duped direction giver had been, actually talking to two different people in the first few minutes of my interview with Castelli? If so, what exactly would that mean regarding human consciousness? Can there be more than one self to a brain? Is there a limit to the number of selves one human brain can be? Would those selves' consciousnesses overlap? Do they *feel* different? How could such a thing happen?

In 1817, SAMUEL LATHAM MITCHILL, a physician, politician, and founding editor of the *Medical Repository,* the first medical journal in the United States, published a strange tale he'd heard from an acquaintance. The friend had told Mitchill about a relative of his, a young lady named Mary Reynolds, who had developed an odd affliction. Already subject to convulsions and having endured a strange episode in which she went blind and deaf for several weeks, only to suddenly regain her faculties, Miss Reynolds one night slept unusually long and deeply. "And when she woke she'd lost every trait of acquired knowledge," according to Mitchill's account. "Her memory was *tabula rasa;* all vestiges, both of words and of things, were obliterated and gone."

When she woke, Reynolds reportedly couldn't recognize family or friends and couldn't read or write, although she learned to do both again quickly. Her nephew, John Reynolds, later wrote that it took her only a day to learn to read again and that once she stopped trying to write from right to left, she learned to write again as well, although not with the beautiful penmanship she'd originally had.

---

* You can see Dr. Simons's tape of his experiment by visiting the Web content area of www.shannonmoffett.com.

No sooner had Reynolds reacquainted herself with her friends and family, the story goes, and relearned a few of her formerly acquired skills than, after another good night's sleep, she woke up restored to her former self. She easily recognized all her old friends, had full mastery of all the skills she'd been working so hard to recapture, and had forgotten the previous few weeks. Everyone apparently gave a big sigh of relief and considered her recovered, but a few weeks later she had another long, deep sleep and woke again to what her family now called her "second state." This switching back and forth continued for years, with Reynolds spending sometimes hours, sometimes days, sometimes weeks, in one state or the other. By the time Mitchill heard the story, her family had long become accustomed to the situation.

Sometime after the first switch, Mary Reynolds's second state seems to have developed a distinct personality of its own, one her nephew called cheery and "even immoderately gay," as opposed to her sober first state. The second personality was — by both her nephew's and other accounts at the time — impetuous, judgmental, mischievous, and either hopelessly naive or a real risk taker. Both the nephew and a family friend wrote of a time when the second-state Reynolds was out walking and saw a rattlesnake, which she didn't seem to recognize as a danger and tried to grab by its tail. Fortunately for her, it escaped into a hole under a log, and she lost her balance, letting go of it. According to her nephew, she then reached into the hole and groped around for the snake, unsuccessfully.

Mitchill's article about Reynolds was the first published in this country on what we'd now call dissociative identity disorder, and was written simply as a case report. There was no discussion of how such a condition might have come about, and Mitchill apparently didn't follow up on Reynolds after printing it. According to her nephew, Reynolds continued to switch back and forth for fifteen years, never sharing memories between the two personalities, until at last she seems to have settled in the second phase and remained there for the last twenty-five years of her life, never again recovering to conscious memory the years she spent in her first state — with one exception. At some point during a second-state phase, Reynolds had a vivid dream of a river and a host of white-robed people listening to a sermon. When she awoke she was still in her second state, but she remembered all the scripture she'd learned while in her first state.

At the time Mitchill wrote about Reynolds, the term *dissociation* hadn't even been coined. It was first used several decades later by the French physician and philosopher Pierre Janet, credited with beginning the modern study of dissociative disorders in the late nineteenth and early twentieth centuries. Janet had planned to study hallucination and perception but was derailed when a mentor introduced him to hypnosis, then known as animal magnetism. He began to study it and other mental phenomena and later used the word *disaggregation* in French (translated to *dissociation* in English) to mean any pathologic mental process disrupting a person's normal sense of a continuous narrative self-history. That definition is essentially the one in use today. According to the fourth edition of the *Diagnostic and Statistical Manual of Mental Disorders,* published by the American Psychiatric Association and the last word in the United States on psychiatric illness: "The essential feature of the Dissociative Disorders is a disruption in the usually integrated functions of consciousness, memory, identity, or perception."

Janet's first experience with dissociation involved a young woman who may have had DID or some other dissociative disorder (the DSM-IV lists five, including "Dissociative Disorder Not Otherwise Specified"), and the case inspired his lifelong fascination with what we would now call the subconscious, what he considered a lower echelon of the mind responsible for certain "automatic" acts, meaning the reasons for them were not consciously available to the person performing them. While Janet never published a fully described theory of that lower echelon and its relation to the conscious mind, as Freud and Jung later did, he strongly believed in its existence and impact on human behavior and regularly used hypnosis and "automatic writing" to confer with his patients' subconscious.

In addition to theorizing about the subconscious, Janet was interested in all manner of dissociative phenomena, and he described cases of what he called "successive existences," which sound, as Mary Reynolds's history does, like examples of what we would today call dissociative identity disorder. Janet believed that dissociative phenomena in general were due to subconscious idées fixes and that such obsessions, and dissociation itself, were associated with prior emotional trauma. He is often credited with having been the first to see a connection between dissociation and trauma, a connection modern experts still maintain is valid.

Along with that legacy, Janet prefigured the later history of the study of dissociation in another way. In an autobiographical essay published toward the end of his career, he wrote that he had spent much of his life struggling for an accord between his scientific inclinations and his early fascination with religion and mysticism, and that studying hypnosis and dissociation had served as a compromise between what he called his "incompatible and diverse tendencies." A century after Janet began his work, dissociation—with DID as its most extreme case—is still straddling the line where science and empiricism butt up against mysticism and the occult.

At that juncture sit people like Judy Castelli. Castelli was raised first in Harrison, New York—a small town where her schoolteachers remembered when her father had attended their classes—and then on Long Island. Her father was a gym instructor and football coach, and then later a guidance counselor and assistant principal. Her mother taught home economics, although she took time off to raise Judy and her two brothers. For most of her adult life,

Castelli told me, "I didn't have an understanding of my childhood as being anything other than 'it was all right.' I didn't think I was really happy, thought I was kind of sad most of my childhood." But she said she had no idea why she would have been sad. When she was sent home by the school psychiatrist from her first year of college because she was suicidally depressed, Castelli still had no idea why she was so sad. This is not unusual, of course: depression usually has no known cause. Neither does schizophrenia, with which she was later diagnosed. At other times, Castelli says, as her symptoms became more bizarre, doctors told her that she had a seizure disorder or that she was malingering.

Schizophrenia is probably the disorder most commonly confused with DID by the general public. The word *schizophrenia* comes from the Greek words for "split" and "mind,"* and to complicate the issue further, people who are eventually diagnosed with DID sometimes spend years, as Castelli did, with a diagnosis of schizophrenia. One of the differences between the two is that, in general, schizophrenics *actually hear* the unreal voices they hallucinate, as if they're coming from outside their heads, the way you'd hear a friend calling you or someone whispering in your ear. People with DID, despite frequently complaining of hearing voices, hear them *inside their heads,* in what Castelli calls "the language of thought." It's a fine distinction, though, and not an easy subtlety to discuss with someone whose voices—whether apparently arising from inside or outside her head—are keeping up a constant chatter.

For whatever reason, in Castelli's case, schizophrenia was the diagnosis that stuck, and so over the next couple of decades, while she was in and out of mental hospitals, while she was cutting herself and burning herself with cigarettes and setting herself on fire, while she

---

*The Greek word from which we've derived the root *phren* referred not only to the mind, but also to the diaphragm, which was once thought to be the seat of the mind.

sometimes talked in funny voices and sometimes heard voices, everyone, including Castelli herself, attributed it to schizophrenia.

Amazingly, during that time Castelli managed to go back to school and then to launch a singing career in Manhattan, where by 1980 she was performing at clubs like the Bottom Line and the legendary but now defunct Folk City. "I was alone at the time," she said. "I was living in a room in somebody's basement, and I had a play going off-Broadway I had written the music for, and I was in that show." She was staying at her manager's apartment in Manhattan during the week to make the commute easier. "It was a crazy, crazy time," she told me. "It was very exciting, and I was just on the brink of having everything work, but I was crazy. Outside of everything else, *I* was crazy."

Around then, Castelli was offered a recording contract by Columbia Records, but the deal fell through when the executive who'd offered it lost his job. Even in the midst of his own catastrophe, he was encouraging. "He said, 'If you can hang in there, you'll have your deal,'" she said. "But I couldn't. That was the thing, you know." Castelli, whose mental health had plummeted as her career began to take off, had become convinced she was worthless, that God wanted her dead. "I could barely take care of myself," she told me, "so when it didn't happen, when the music deal didn't happen, when the record didn't even happen, it was almost a relief that I could say, 'OK, now I can stop,' you know? Now I can just do something else. And I decided to do art and taught myself to do stained glass."

Still in and out of mental hospitals, Castelli couldn't hold a job and was living in friends' apartments, just on the border of homelessness. It was at a Halloween party at one of those apartments that she met Phyllis, who later became her companion. Phyllis was an actress and physical-education teacher who happened to have built a house in the Hamptons in the seventies, when such a thing could be done on a gym teacher's salary.

Soon after meeting Phyllis, Castelli was asked to leave the

apartment where she was staying. But now, she told me, "I knew Phyllis had this house in East Hampton, and I said, 'Nobody's living in your house,' because she lived in Manhattan then. 'Could I live there?' And she said, 'Ooooh, OK!' So that's pretty much how we became friends, and then, you know, and then we became more than friends, and we've been together ever since."

The arrangement they made two decades ago turned out to have been good for both of them. Phyllis, a stocky woman with a salt-and-pepper bob and a merry, booming laugh, told me, "She wasn't so scary or had terrible symptoms or was violent or anything like that." Their meeting began a more joyful time in Phyllis's life and a more stable time in Castelli's. Although Castelli was still, as she herself put it, "totally nuts," she began going to a therapist she liked and got a job at a day-treatment center for the mentally ill, where she had once been a patient. There she taught other patients to make stained-glass lampshades, which, in the entrepreneurial spirit characteristic of Castelli, they sold to Bloomingdale's.

For the next few years, Castelli was feeling better and held the job at the day-treatment center. She said it was one day while at work there that she suddenly felt particularly bad—bad in a way she can only describe by saying she knew she was "so not OK." According to Castelli, she called her therapist, who told her to come in on her lunch hour. Once Castelli had arrived, her therapist asked her what was wrong, and Castelli said she didn't know, at which point her therapist asked her if maybe there was some other part of Castelli that knew. Which was when Castelli heard the word "torture" in a deep, raspy voice and realized the word had come out of her own mouth. It was the first appearance, as far as she knows, of the alter identity she calls Gravelly Voice. The rest of that session is hazy and fragmented in Castelli's memory, or at least the memory accessible to any of the alters I spoke with. Later, another persona appeared that Castelli has named the One Who Would Set Us on Fire; he was obsessed with burning his/Castelli's body. He was one of six other alters who, following Gravelly Voice's example, came out and spoke that day, all sharing tales of childhood abuse that Castelli was suddenly remembering.

At that point, "everything else kind of fell into place," she told me. "As soon as I got the multiple diagnosis, I said, 'Oh, yeah, that explains that, now I get it.'" She was briefly admitted to a hospital specializing in dissociative disorders, but when she was released, she paradoxically felt more comfortable with herself and her life than ever before. She says she still isn't "normal," though. I asked her how exactly she's different from those of us she calls "singletons." OK, so she had been more nervous and wary when we met in the driveway, and more relaxed and ready to talk when we were in her house and had chatted for a while. Don't we all show different faces to the world? What makes my faces simply the facets of one personality and her faces entirely different people?

"I'm gonna switch because that'll be easier," she said. "Just before you came, I was saying to Phyllis—" she broke off to explain, "I'm also Judy, but I'm a different one—I'm younger than her," which was hardly necessary. This Judy had a radically different manner of speech from the two I'd heard until then. Where the others were fluent and adult sounding—the most recent a rapid talker with a bouncy cadence—this one was childlike, slow and careful and plaintive. As she spoke, Castelli curled her whole body in around herself, somehow managing to look up at me despite being taller by several inches. Putting the thumb of one hand and the middle finger of another together, she twisted her hands so that alternately the opposite thumb and middle finger touched, "Itsy-Bitsy Spider" style. "So I was saying to her," this little Judy said, "that she's coming now, she's coming, the lady, and we don't know what she's gonna say, we don't know what she wants us to say, we don't know what she's doing, what is she *doing*? Phyllis said, 'Don't worry about it, it'll be OK, it'll be fine. You'll do good.'" The child Judy gave a little giggle, and then she switched back while still talking to me. "I'm still switching, my voice is not quite as little as it was, but I'm sort of going back to who I was. So there it was," she said, and was fully back in the physicality and voice of what she calls a Big Judy.

Oh, boy. Castelli later told me how frustrating it is to appear on talk shows, something she says she's done several times in order to educate the public about DID so that sufferers get earlier and more appropriate treatment than she did. "On radio and TV," she told me, "they really want to see it or hear it. They're looking for that. They want to be able to say, 'This is what happens'" when a person with DID switches to an alter identity. "But then you get this reaction that, 'Oh, that's acting. I can do that, too,' you know?" She laughed. "So it's like you're caught between a rock and a hard place. If I switch, they say, 'I can do that,' or 'She made that up,' or 'Oh, yeah, yeah, I can talk like a four-year-old, too.'"

Which I have to admit pretty much covers what I was thinking when confronted with the bizarrely unsettling sight of a fifty-three-year-old woman referring to me as a lady in a pitch-perfect embodiment of a child's fear-tinged respect for unfamiliar adults. However realistic her behavior, the young Judy seemed fake, horribly fake. But how could a child's mannerisms performed by an adult body not? What if you could somehow put the brain of a kindergartner in the body of a middle-aged woman—would the gestures and turns of phrase she used seem more genuine than those a talented and observant actor could perform? And wouldn't she eventually grow up? Could this little Judy possibly be real, frozen in the never-never land of Castelli's consciousness?

IN 1977, SEVENTEEN years before Castelli's alters appeared, a young Sally Field starred in the made-for-TV movie *Sybil*, based on the story of a real woman diagnosed with what was then known as multiple personality disorder. The movie was wildly popular and won two

Emmy Awards, but it portrayed a disorder then considered vanishingly rare. There had been only a handful of reported cases in this country in the century and a half since Mitchill's account of Mary Reynolds.

Sybil's airing was followed three years later (and not coincidentally, some say) by the inclusion of multiple personality disorder in the third edition of the *Diagnostic and Statistical Manual,* giving the illness official recognition in the eyes of the nation's psychiatrists. In the fourth edition of the DSM, which came out in 1994, the year Castelli was diagnosed with the illness, its name was changed to dissociative identity disorder by a panel of experts that included Dr. David Spiegel, a psychiatrist and professor at Stanford University whom I visited after meeting Castelli.

Spiegel is a mild-mannered man who wears an enormous stainless-steel watch on his wrist and a cell phone clipped to his belt at all times, but he spared me half an hour to talk about DID. He gave me his complete attention during that time, lolling back in his chair with one foot up on his desk, drinking coffee from a thermos and ignoring his ringing phone and the tones announcing incoming e-mail that emanated from his computer every minute or two.

I first asked Spiegel about current DID research, which is practically nonexistent. In fact, the scientific literature on the disorder hasn't gotten much more informative since Mitchill described Mary Reynolds's case. Since then, there have been about four well-known cases of DID in this country: "Miss Beauchamp," described by Morton Prince in 1906; "Eve," described by Thigpen and Cleckley in 1957; "Sibyl," described by Cornelia Wilbur and Flora Rheta Schreiber in the book on which the movie was based; and Truddi Chase, who wrote a memoir of her own experience with DID, published in 1987. The published scientific work on dissociative identity disorder essentially consists of these and a few other case studies. There has apparently been only one report of an fMRI study on the subject, in 1999, and the experiment was small scale at best. It involved only one subject, a woman who, after years of therapy, had learned—as Castelli has—to control her switching from alter to alter. The investigators asked her to switch repeatedly between one of her adult alters and a child alter named Guardian. They also, as a control, had her *imagine* switching between the adult alter and an imaginary child personality named Player. They were looking solely for what happened during the switch, though, rather than for differences in active brain areas from one personality to the next.

They found that each switch was accompanied by a change in activation in the hippocampus and medial temporal lobe. The woman's hippocampus was also smaller than normal, but post-traumatic stress disorder, with which she'd also been diagnosed, is known to cause a smaller-than-normal hippocampus. Dissociative identity disorder, as it's understood today, seems to arise from chronic trauma and stress, so it is unlikely that it will ever be easy to determine whether a DID sufferer's small hippocampus is due to DID or to the trauma. But it does seem as if fMRI could be used to answer some of the obvious questions about DID, such as whether there is a particular brain-activation pattern for an individual alter, or whether each of a subject's alters—many of which don't share memories with other alters—has access to only a part of the hippocampus. Yet no one has used fMRI to try to answer those questions.

I asked Spiegel why. "You know, these studies take big money, and it's hard to get the funding," he said. "Unlike other parts of psychiatry—where people will argue about the nature of the symptoms or how biologically based they are or something—with this there are people that claim it doesn't exist, and that it's a creation of inept or malicious therapists who look for the symptoms and find them wherever they look."

Scholars who doubt the existence of DID as a legitimate psychiatric disorder are plentiful and come in a variety of flavors. All of them point to the leap in diagnosed cases in the last couple of decades as evidence for their views. Since *Sybil*'s release and multiple personality disorder's inclusion in the DSM, diagnoses of the disorder in this country have skyrocketed. No one is quite sure how many cases there are at present in the United States, but most guesses put the number in the thousands. Some scoffers think those claiming to suffer from DID are out-and-out malingerers, with the payoff for the fakers being attention, the benefits of the sick role, and relief from having to take responsibility for their actions. They point to DID's use as a legal defense and argue that it's a mighty convenient way for a criminal to avoid the consequences of his or her crimes.

Other skeptics, while not completely doubting the existence of the disorder, believe it exists only as a metaphor for internal states, basically another way of talking about moods. In their view, patients aren't exactly playacting but somehow create DID within themselves in an attempt to understand why their lives are difficult, and the different alters are really just new names for what we would call "angry," "sad," "deliriously happy," and so on.

It's a tempting idea and fits, in some ways, with what Castelli told me about what it's like to be her. Or them. While visiting her, I had asked if the alter I was speaking to had different moods. "Hmmm," she said, after a pause in which she looked slightly puzzled. "I think we're more likely to switch to someone else, rather than have a couple of levels of emotion or something in one. Yeah, I think we kind of— I think we switch to somebody that *does* that better." She gave the example of the Worrier, a male alter of hers whose job is to worry. "A lot of the worrying gets taken care of by that one personality," she said, and then explained what she sees as the distinction between when the rest of us worry and when she does. "So *you* kind of—you go into a worried moment or a worried state, or you're just going to be worried for three days. It's on your mind, but you're still you. And I think that's the difference. If I switch to the Worrier, that's ALL Worrier does is worry—that's all he knows how to do. So there's no way to comfort that, there's no way to move out of that, unless I move to another personality."

Who exactly the "I" is that would move to another personality is vague. When I asked if there was a sort of master Judy, she said, "I don't know who would be the host Judy, who would be the biggest, the one that everybody reports to. I couldn't tell you. I assume right now it's me."

Other doubters of the legitimacy of DID back up their position by pointing out that hypnosis is often used in both the diagnosis and the treatment of DID, arguing that the alters and the illness itself could easily be the result of hypnotic suggestion in susceptible patients seeking mental-health care for other problems. They point out that psychiatrists and social workers are only human, and that either by design (in order to make a name for themselves as specialists in an area full of publicity opportunities) or unconscious bias (influenced by the media), they may lead their patients to exhibit the symptoms of DID. The fact— acknowledged by those who believe in DID— that people with the disorder have been shown to be significantly more hypnotizable than the general population gives credence to such skeptics' views.

There is some other evidence, although not much and certainly not conclusive, to support the theory that DID is hypnotically induced. Dr. Nicholas Spanos, an expert in hypnosis and a professor of psychology at Carleton University in Ottawa until his death in 1994, ran an experiment that he believed showed that DID could be hypnotically induced. The experiment was inspired by the case of Kenneth Bianchi, known as the Hillside Strangler, who used multiple personality disorder as a defense in his trial. When Bianchi was apprehended, he was given a psychiatric evaluation that included hypnosis. The examining psychiatrist and Bianchi's defense team believed Bianchi's behavior under hypnosis showed he had a hidden personality named Steve, and that Steve was responsible for the murders.

Bianchi's evaluation was videotaped and transcribed, and Spanos, after reviewing it, hypothesized that the session could actually have helped Bianchi fake DID or even believe he suffered from it. To test his theory, Spanos recruited a group of undergraduate students and asked them to participate in a role-playing experiment in which each would act the part of a murderer on trial. He divided the students into three groups, the first of which was given what he called the Bianchi treatment. The members of that group were initially asked who they were (to which they were to respond with either "Harry" or "Betty"), then hypnotized and addressed with a monologue "taken almost verbatim from the Bianchi interview," Spanos wrote in the paper describing his experiment. For instance, "I've talked a bit to Harry (Betty) but I think perhaps there might be another part of Harry (Betty) that I haven't talked to, another part that maybe feels somewhat differently from the part that I've talked to. And I would like to communicate with that other part."

Spanos's researchers spoke directly to the subject's "Part" and asked it to lift the "accused's" hand to signal its presence. Regardless of the subjects' response, they were asked, "Part, are you the same thing as Harry (Betty) or are you different in any way?" The Part was then asked other questions, including who it was, if it had a name that it could be called by, and what Harry (or Betty) was like.

The students in the second group were also initially asked who they were and then hypnotized and given a little speech about the complexity of personality and how some thoughts may be blocked off from the conscious mind, "almost like there are different people inside of us with different feelings and ideas." These subjects were then again asked who they were, if they had a name they could be called by, and so forth. The members of the third group were asked to identify themselves as Harry or Betty. They were not hypnotized but were given the same speech as the second group.

At a second session, each subject was given two identical questionnaires. The members of the two hypnotized groups were hypnotized again, and if they'd adopted a separate identity under hypnosis, that identity was called out and asked to fill out the questionnaire. They were then told that upon awakening, they would be Harry or Betty once more, and when awake, they were asked to fill out the questionnaire again as either Harry or Betty. The members of the group who had not been hypnotized in the first session were not hypnotized in the second but were simply asked to complete the questionnaire twice in a row.

In the end, ten of the sixteen students who received the Bianchi treatment were judged to have taken on a different identity from the Harry/Betty identity, while three of the second group and none of the third group had done so. In students who had assumed an alternate identity, that identity gave dramatically different answers on the questionnaires from those given by the Harry (Betty) identity. The questionnaire consisted of sentence-completion questions about mothers, anger, sexual thoughts, and self-perception, and one subject, for instance, filled in a sentence beginning "My mother is" with "a scum bag probably just like yours" under hypnosis, but then wrote "a clean, very good woman" once awake and playing the role of Harry.

Spanos's use of hypnosis in his study was interesting because, as with DID, few can agree on what hypnosis is. Unlike DID, however, hypnosis is generally accepted among clinicians and scientists as a valid phenomenon, which is surprising in light of the fact that few studies have shown any measurable and reproducible physiologic differences between people's bodies and brains when they're hypnotized and when they're awake. In addition, there has been at least one study demonstrating that even hypnosis experts presented with an intermingled group of hypnotized and pretending-to-be-hypnotized subjects can't tell the difference. Nevertheless, there have been many studies showing that people both feel different and behave differently when hypnotized, and that interventions performed while subjects are hypnotized will make a bigger difference in their subsequent behavior than if the same interventions are performed on subjects who are awake.

I asked Spiegel, who studies hypnosis and uses it in his practice, how he would define the term. "Well," he said, "it can be understood as a state of highly focused attention with a suspension of peripheral awareness. So it's like—have you ever been so caught up in a good movie you forgot you were watching a movie?" That sensation, he said, is basically the same as being hypnotized. So for people who are thus caught up, "it's not that they couldn't figure out it was a fantasy, but for the moment they're just *in* the imagined world, and so what happens to the hero is really happening, and they get scared. And then when it's over, they say, 'Oh, yeah, that was just a movie.' You know, the playwrights call that the suspension of disbelief." That state, he says, "allows people to do things they don't ordinarily do, so they can experience less control in parts of their body, or they can actually enhance control, they can reduce pain—" He broke off to show me the results of a study he did in collaboration with a researcher at Harvard. The two explored color perception in subjects under hypnosis and collected data showing that when people envision nonexistent color differences under hypnosis, "they actually change blood flow in the color-processing portions of the brain." Spiegel's study was a functional-imaging study, but it used positron-emission-tomography instead of fMRI. Like fMRI, PET relies on detecting the difference in blood flow to active and nonactive regions of the brain. Spiegel pulled up an image from the study on his monitor.

"This is the occipital cortex," he said, pointing at the picture. "This is the back of the head; the occipital cortex is where we process vision." He then pointed out the lingual and fusiform gyri, "where blood flow increases when you're looking at color compared to black and white."*

For the experiment, Spiegel and his collaborators took eight highly hypnotizable Harvard students (who were otherwise normal—

---

* The color-processing region of the fusiform gyrus is separate from the fusiform face area.

another argument Spiegel likes to give against the DID doubters is that there are plenty of highly hypnotizable people around who don't have DID) and showed them two patterns of rectangles made up of smaller rectangles.

In one of the patterns, the rectangles were filled in with bright colors, while the other was made up only of gray boxes, with different shades for each rectangle.

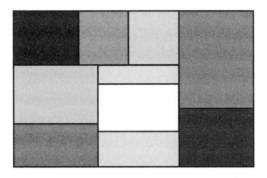

The subjects were shown each of the images four times — twice under hypnosis and twice without being hypnotized. Both under hypnosis and not, one of the two times they were shown the grayscale pattern, they were asked to visualize it in color. They were also asked to visualize the colored pattern as black and white, once while under hypnosis and once without being hypnotized. In all cases their brain activity was recorded via PET as they were shown the images.

As you'd expect, both hypnotized and nonhypnotized subjects' color-processing areas were active when they looked at the colored pattern, and showed decreased activity when they looked at the black-and-white pattern. In the case of the nonhypnotized trials, subjects' brains reflected what was actually in front of them, even when they were trying to see the colored pattern as black and white or the grayscale pattern as colored. But while hypnotized and trying to "see" the black and white image as colored, subjects demonstrated "a significant increase in blood flow in the color-processing region of the brain," Spiegel told me. "When they're looking at color but think it's black and white, there's a significant decrease in blood flow." Under hypnosis, he said, it appears that "believing is seeing."

Clearly, the students in Spanos's study didn't actually believe they had DID, despite the hypnotic intervention. And it isn't particularly surprising that the interviews that focused on the concept of compartmentalized personalities were more likely to plant the idea of using multiple personality disorder as a defense in the minds of role-playing college kids who had to keep up the act for only a few hours. But Spanos's paper is often cited in the contentious debate over dissociative identity disorder as evidence that the illness is a figment of the imagination of either patient or therapist.

As a result of the confusion and acrimony surrounding the disorder, said Spiegel, "there are very few NIH research grants on dissociative disorders per se, because the kind of people that like doing research tend to be smart enough not to try to do research on this." And, he added, "when people put in grants, they often don't fare well in review committees because someone will say, 'Not only is it a bad design, but the disorder doesn't even exist, so it's not worth spending any money on.'"

I asked Spiegel whether he and the psychiatric community had changed the name from multiple personality disorder to dissociative identity disorder to evade some of the controversy surrounding the illness. No, he said. He believes the latter term more accurately describes the illness as "a failure of integration of aspects of identity, memory, and consciousness, not a proliferation of personalities." In those with DID, some portions of the mind won't be able to tolerate feeling angry, he said, and "others can't tolerate feeling vulnerable or sad, so if something bad happens they say, 'Well, it happened to her.

It didn't happen to me.'" So, as he likes to say, the problem with people like Castelli "is not that they have more than one personality but that they have *less* than one personality."

Nevertheless, in addition to the increase in diagnoses of DID in recent years, there has been a recorded increase in the number of alter identities per diagnosis. When multiple personality disorder was first recognized and described in modern times, the average number of identities per case was two or three. Today, many patients, like Castelli, have more than that, and some patients and their psychiatrists claim to have identified hundreds of alters. Skeptics use that fact as further reason to doubt the validity of DID as a genuine disorder, arguing that such an increase can only be due to patients' or their therapists' trying to outfragment other cases.

"Some people are unduly credulous, and I've seen therapists who will play games on the floor with child alters and have them sit on their lap, which is *wrong*," Spiegel said when I raised that argument. "Once I've determined that they have a dissociative disorder, and I sort of know who the main players are in their personality structure, I start losing interest in how many personalities I can stumble across. It'll happen anyway, but I don't map them and I don't count them and all that; and I do think that there is a danger that if you get too interested in it, the patient'll go, 'Oh, OK, he wants more personalities. I'll see what I can do.'"

Spiegel has an interesting take on whether therapists might be implanting DID. Castelli told me she had wondered if maybe she had DID years before being diagnosed with it and had even asked her therapist if she might have it. According to Castelli, her therapist said, "No, Judy, you don't want to be multiple. Being schizophrenic is hard enough." She also told Castelli, "You don't want to be multiple. They can't really *do* anything with multiples." Which Spiegel believes is often the attitude of therapists.

"Are there therapists that see it under every rock? Yeah, there are," he said. But not many. "There are a lot more doctors who either don't know about it, or who *do* know about it and think it's a farce and tell patients, 'You don't have this.' And it doesn't go away." He told me that on average it takes six years from the time the first symptoms appear until the time a patient is diagnosed with DID. During that time, he pointed out, "You can be sure they've seen plenty of people who say, 'I don't know what this is, but make it go away,' or 'It doesn't exist,' or 'You've got something else,' or whatever—and it doesn't disappear. So if suggestion did it, it oughta work in both directions, and it *doesn't*. There's something wrong with these people." He argues that the reason that there are more cases of DID diagnosed today than ever before is that more therapists know something about the illness and how to differentiate it from schizophrenia, and that more patients are willing to seek psychiatric help today than in the past.

A COUPLE OF DAYS after I first met Castelli, I sat down with Phyllis while Castelli was taking a nap. Now that I had spent some time with them, it made more sense to me that Phyllis would have agreed so readily to let a mentally ill homeless woman she barely knew live in her house. Raised Jewish in Brooklyn, Phyllis, who has since died of breast cancer, had a steadfastly practical outlook and a bit of the earth mother about her that must have made her want to take care of Castelli. But she also had a comic streak that garnered her improv roles on Conan O'Brien's show, and Castelli—or many of her identities, especially the children—has a bubbly, infectious charm and a fresh way of looking at things that must have appealed to that part of Phyllis.

When I asked her what it was like to live with Castelli, Phyllis said, "Well, let's just say it's interesting." According to her, although the adult Judys usually keep a tight leash on her child alters ("I'm very strict with them," a Big Judy told me), they occasionally come out unbidden. For instance, they once attended a friend's dinner party. "One of the fellas there was a story teller for the New York City school system," Phyllis told me. At the other guests' behest, the man began telling one of his stories. "And he was telling it like he would to a third-grade class, and we were all very amused," she said. All except Castelli. "Judy's little girl came out and asked questions, you know, like a child would: 'And what else did he do?'"

Castelli had told me that walking past the toy department in a store is often hard for her, as she can feel her child alters tugging at her to let them go play. Phyllis gave another example: "When there's a circus—we have a lot of little circuses that come around here, and I *know* that as soon as we go by, one of the little ones is going to come out and say, 'Can we go?'"

And?

"And we've gone, you know, and it's been great. See, I'm a child, too, basically, and it just works very well for us." However, there are unique difficulties in living with a multiple. For instance, despite the fact that Castelli used to be a singer, Phyllis told me that occasionally the two will be out and someone will ask Castelli to sing for them, "and she'll tell me that the one who can sing is not here." That's not the only skill that appears to have become inaccessible. One of the Judys used to do the couple's cooking, Phyllis said, but "we haven't seen her in, like, a year."

Castelli says such amnesias are a source of much frustration for her. When I visited them, she and Phyllis were just packing up to go back to Tucson, where they spend half the year, and Castelli was trying to figure out what art supplies to take with her. She had planned to do some wood inlay, one of the crafts she taught herself after quitting singing. But in trying to figure out what to take with her, she discovered that she no longer knew how. She had done at least eight pieces and had gotten fairly skilled before she stopped. "So somebody had a good time with it," she said, "but it didn't filter to me. So unless that part just wants to come out and take over when we're actually standing at the saw, then I guess it's up to me, and I'll do the best I can." Given what we know about nondeclarative memory, it would be interesting to see if, like HM, she would in fact be capable of doing the work once she had the tools in her hands. But meanwhile, she said, "it's like I'm starting over."

If Castelli can somehow have parts of her mind—richly experiential parts—walled off from other parts' experience, what does it mean about our brains' supposedly integrated capacity for consciousness? Robert Stickgold himself—whose wife is a clinical psychologist specializing in dissociative disorders—pointed out to me that DID could be evidence for the philosopher's side in the argument over the fusiform gyrus's capacity for independent experience. We don't know how Castelli's divisions are maintained within her mind—whether they're based on anatomy or neuronal connections or something else. There are plenty of people who would say the divisions don't exist at all, but many of those can't quite bring themselves to call DID sufferers liars, in which case they must admit that those with DID *believe* some parts of their minds can't remember events accessible to other parts. What is the difference between believing you can't consciously remember something and not remembering it?

AMONG THOSE WHO BELIEVE in DID, it's generally agreed that Pierre Janet was right about psychological trauma's causing the phenomenon. Particularly correlated with the development of DID is long-term chronic trauma sustained before the age of about nine years old, the sort associated with physical abuse of a child by a family member, the sort Castelli, that day in her therapist's office, found herself remembering having experienced at the hands of someone she will only identify as a female caretaker.

Such an association is difficult to demonstrate clearly, however. For unclear reasons, DID is usually not diagnosed until the third or fourth decade of life, years after the abuse would have occurred. It's hard to prove or disprove an accusation of child abuse, even when made while the victim is still a child, given the obstacles to obtaining a good history, the lack of corroborating witnesses, and the difficulty of differentiating between abuse-related injuries and the normal scrapes and bruises of childhood. The task can be impossible when the alleged abuse happened decades earlier, the physical signs have disappeared, and both the victims and the perpetrators have grown older and have layered their memories under years of denial. In the case of alleged abuse victims with DID, often the only thing researchers have to work with is the say-so of people who are literally crazy.

In addition, many with DID seem to have repressed their memories of abuse for years, a symptom that adds to DID's suspect nature. We all have things we'd rather not remember, the argument goes—things we try not to think about and turn away from when they do float into our consciousness. If we were asked questions about those things, we might not *want* to answer, but we *could.* Those memories are there, whether we like them or not. Truly forgetting them would be impossible. Forgetting is simply not voluntary.

Or is it? Not long after I visited Castelli, John Gabrieli's name popped up in the news. His lab had conducted a study in which subjects were given a list of pairs of unrelated words (for instance, *ordeal* and *roach*) and instructed to memorize them. The participants were then placed in an fMRI scanner and given a succession of single words from the pairs. Before each word was given, subjects were instructed either to attempt to think of its associated word or to try *not* to think of the associated word, to prevent it from entering their minds for the four seconds that its partner word was displayed. As a basis for comparison, some of the word pairs the subjects had memorized never appeared at all during the scanning.

Later, subjects were brought back and again asked to provide the other word when shown single words from each of the pairs they had learned. On the whole, participants had the best recall for words from pairs they'd actively tried to remember in the previous trial. They did significantly worse on the pairs that hadn't been brought up on the first recall test, which makes sense, since those words would have been less fresh in their minds. But subjects scored even worse on the words they had actively tried to suppress — far worse than on the words they had attempted to recall during the first test, and significantly worse than on the words that weren't brought up at all during the first test. They did so poorly on recalling the previously suppressed words, in fact, that even much more direct clues than their associated words (for instance, being given the word *insect* to prompt them to remember *roach*) often didn't help them call up the words they'd tried to keep out of their minds during the first test.

The fMRI data, unsurprisingly, showed less hippocampal activity during the trials in which subjects tried to block the memory of a word than in those in which they tried to remember it. When subjects actively tried not to remember a word, however, the scanner showed increased activity in the lateral prefrontal cortex. The lateral prefrontal cortex is an area believed to be important in executive functioning, meaning it helps keep us from saying what we think in circumstances where we deem it detrimental to our success, or from following through when anger makes us raise our hands to hit someone.

In addition to providing evidence for our apparent ability to suppress memories, Gabrieli's study yielded another surprising finding. As you might expect, the more hippocampal activity present while subjects actively tried to remember a word on the first test, the more likely the subject was to recall the word on the later test. But increased hippocampal activity during the trials in which subjects were asked to suppress their memories corresponded to decreased ability to recall the suppressed word on the second test. Gabrieli and his colleagues hypothesized that in those cases, the increased blood flow to the hippocampus might represent spontaneous intrusions of the memory of the word as subjects tried to block it out. They proposed that those intrusions might have resulted in the need for increased executive control to overcome them, ultimately leading to increased forgetting.

They interpreted their findings to mean that the act of suppressing a memory is an active one, under voluntary control, and pointed out that their work bears on the long-standing debate in psychiatric circles and society at large over whether that's possible. "Whether suppression can produce complete and lasting amnesia for an unwanted memory," they wrote, "remains unknown. However, this work confirms the existence of an active process by which people can prevent awareness of an unwanted past experience and specifies the neural systems that underlie it. This process causes forgetting. Thus, the current findings provide the first neurobiological model of the voluntary form of repression proposed by Freud, a model that integrates this otherwise controversial proposal with widely accepted and fundamental mechanisms for controlling behavior."

The question of whether such suppressed memories can subsequently be recalled will have to await further research. And many would deny that forgetting a word on a short-term, low-stakes test in which the memories lack important associations is evidence that something as important, chronic, and deeply experiential as long-term abuse can be forgotten. Even Castelli says she is plagued by her own skepticism and wonders sometimes if DID really exists or if she was ever really abused at all ("You have *doubt*, you know?"). For the rest of us, it's much easier to believe both DID and recovered memories of child abuse are made up. It's much more comfortable—that way, we don't have to think about someone's hurting a child or confront tough questions about memory, selfhood, and the unified and individual nature of a human consciousness. We don't have to try to conceive the inconceivable: the idea of more than one consciousness seated in a single human brain.

And yet sometimes the inconceivable happens. In 1997, Dr. Dorothy Otnow Lewis, a professor of psychiatry at New York University, published the results of a study of prison inmates with dissociative identity disorder. For the project, she had reviewed the objective evidence of past child abuse suffered by prisoners on death row who met the four DSM criteria for dissociative identity disorder, which are (a) that patients have two or more identities or personality states, which (b) recurrently take control of the person's behavior, leading to (c) an inability to recall personal information so great that it couldn't be attributed to ordinary forgetfulness, and that (d) the disturbance is not due to physiologic effects of a substance or other medical condition. There had been extensive investigation into these men's lives in the course of the legal proceedings against them, and Lewis was able to take advantage of a collection of data that couldn't have been gathered without the resources available to the prosecution and defense in a murder trial.

One of the men she described in her study was an inmate who'd bounced around from foster home to foster home before committing a murder and ending up in prison. This man had at least one alter that was a woman, who liked to wear dresses and put sanitary napkins in her underwear. An array of evidence from doctors' visits and social services reports from his childhood shows that when he as a little boy, his mother abused him so hideously and bizarrely that just thinking about it makes you want to shut down your own mind. She regularly locked him in the closet, whether to punish him or just to get him out of the way is unclear. She pulled both his thumbs out of their sockets. And she also habitually tied him down and gave him enemas that she told him contained blood, then inserted tampons into his rectum to soak up the liquid.

Another man had been used, when he was a boy, as an actor in child-pornography movies produced by his father and uncle. When he was uncooperative, someone punished him by forcing the child to sit down on a hot stove burner. In his case, the burn scars on his perineum served as additional documentation of the abuse.

Yet another man's caretakers had seen fit to punish him, at two years old, by pouring scalding water on his penis. They later tried to "circumcise" the little boy at home.

These are only the atrocities for which legally acceptable documentation is available. As Lewis wrote, "The term 'abuse' does not do justice to the quality of mistreatment these individuals endured. A more accurate term would be 'torture.'" Ongoing torture, with no possibility for escape, not even the hope of rescue, as the people who ought to have been the rescuers were themselves the torturers.

Once we've accepted the existence of such unthinkable abominations and the miracle that some of those tormented children do survive, is it really so incredible that they might have found an extraordinary coping mechanism? Neuroscientists have only recently begun to recognize how dramatically our brains can reorganize when necessary. This capacity, known as plasticity, allows for phenomena such as the one Roberta Glick alluded to regarding an infant's brain's ability to regain full function even after major damage. Such recovery happens not (or not primarily) by healing and the regeneration of damaged areas, but by the redistribution of duties among the neurons left intact. While our brains lose much of their plasticity as we exit childhood, even in adulthood they maintain a remarkable ability to adapt to injury or new experience. The neurologist V. S. Ramachandran, for instance, has demonstrated that after the amputation of an arm, touching the face of the amputee will activate areas in the brain that were once devoted solely to sensory experience of the arm. Rather than lying fallow when no longer receiving sensory input from the arm, those neurons reorganized to respond to tactile stimulation of an area still capable of sending signals to the brain. Other researchers have shown that when volunteers are taught to read Braille using their left hand, the amount of brain space in the sensory cortex dedicated to that hand increases, a change detectible after only a few days of training. Such juggling of neurons' responsibilities isn't limited to occurring within one sensory modality—blind people's brains have been shown to reorganize so that the occipital cortex, once dedicated to processing signals from the retina, is instead used for processing sound. While this can happen in adulthood, the young (prepubertal) human brain apparently has an extraordinary capacity for such restructuring.

Which brings us back to dissociative identity disorder. Anyone who's ever spaced out in a boring lecture or while waiting in line at the bank knows it's possible to avoid at least mild unpleasantness by going away inside one's head. Is it so impossible that a child, given no other choice, might learn to do such a thing to avoid overwhelming pain and shame? And that once such going away became a habit, a name might be given to the mental place where she went? Once enormous portions of a child's life were spent in that mental place, mightn't it become as much a part of herself as the mental place from which she'd fled? Somehow the brain would have to set up barriers to allow true escape, at least until it was necessary to call up information available only in the first mental place. Eventually, maybe switching back and forth from mental place to mental place would be easy, effortless, unconscious. And then, with some information available in one place and some in another, a third might be created to avoid the pain that was accumulating in the second place. Such plasticity in higher-order processing has yet to be documented experimentally, in part because we don't really understand yet—as we are beginning to with sensory pathways—where such processing happens.

. . .

WHEN I VISITED HIM, I asked Spiegel about recovered memories. "That's a very complex area," he said, "but my general take on it is that if it's possible to have a false memory that abuse occurred when it didn't, it's also possible to have a false memory that abuse didn't occur when it did, which is what people with dissociative disorders tend to have. And there are three million cases of childhood sexual or physical abuse every year in this country; one million come to attention somehow. So you know, for every case where somebody's falsely accused when it didn't happen, there must be a lot of cases where they're not accused when it did. But of course, the whole notion of childhood sexual abuse is so—so awful that it tends to arouse passions."

He attributes some of the disbelief in DID and science's lack of progress toward understanding the illness to those passions. "I still find it puzzling or disappointing that there's such a low order of discourse about this disorder," he said. "We have all kinds of disagreements about schizophrenia and what causes it, and we don't believe the delusions of the schizophrenic, but we don't say schizophrenia doesn't exist; we just say they have delusions. We're not sure what causes them, and there's disagreement about it, but it's legitimate disagreement. But somehow with dissociation, you know, it's a different kind of discussion." His goal is to steer the field toward higher ground. "I think the discourse has to be more research-driven and more empirical and more dispassionate," he said.

Castelli agrees. "You know, science is wonderful," she once said to me. Even in what little research has been done on DID, she said, "they're actually able to show changes in the brain and in the body" of people with DID, which she finds helpful in the face of so much doubt. Somehow, seeing physical changes is oddly reassuring, providing a sense that something "really is" going on. The idea is a strange holdover from the time before we had truly begun to grapple with Crick's astonishing hypothesis. Such artifacts are all around. As Stickgold told me, "People will say, 'Oh, no, that's not psychological;

there's something *happening* in your *brain*.'" And Castelli said, "There's so many disbelievers that say, 'Oh, yeah, it's all in your head.'" To which she says, "Yeah, thank you very much. Yeah, I get that."

When Castelli was hospitalized immediately after being diagnosed with DID, she arrived on a Friday night. "It was horrible," she said. "I was all over the place, I was switching left and right, and I was having memories left and right, and there was nobody, really, coming around and helping, almost. It felt like, 'Why did I do this,' you know? 'So why am I here?'" But then Monday came and the psychiatrists returned to work. "When I did see the psychiatrist, I said, 'How is this supposed to work?'" According to Castelli, the psychiatrist told her to keep a journal, to ask who needed to talk and then let them. "And that's what I did," says Castelli. "I started the top of the page every time with 'Who needs to talk?' And somebody always answered."

It was through her journals that the parts of Castelli I spoke with said they learned why she'd been setting herself on fire. It turned out that the One Who Would Set Us on Fire was a little boy. He wrote in the journal, "I will set me on fire as big as the sky and the angels will see, and the angels will say, 'I see, I see.'" "So his job at that moment," Castelli told me, "was to show the angels that we were in that kind of pain, and what better way to do it but to set yourself on fire, set the body on fire, and let it just be a big flame and big smoke and everybody should see. It goes beyond cry for help. You talk about magical thinking—I have a lot of parts that do that magical kind of thinking."

Somehow I hadn't pictured the fire setter as a little boy. In fact, most of Castelli's alters turned out to be less frightening than I'd imagined. Before meeting her, I had read a little about Castelli on her Web site,* which she set up to serve as an information source about DID and the journal writing that she feels helped her deal with the illness.

---

* The address is http://www.multiple-personality.com.

Reading there about Gravelly Voice saying "torture" in her therapist's office reminded me so much of the little boy saying "redrum" in the movie of Stephen King's *The Shining* that I found it hard not to imagine Castelli's head as a sort of Overlook Hotel with an ax-brandishing Jack Nicholson on the prowl, whom I somehow equated with Gravelly Voice.

But when I asked Castelli about him, she said, "Yeah, he's the speaker of truth, Gravelly Voice." She went on: "We think of him as the most courageous, the most fearless, because he's the one that said 'torture' out loud first. That was like the biggest gift, you know?"

At the end of our first interview, Castelli, in a persona whose name I never got, but whom I'll call the Demonstrator, showed me some of her artwork. The Demonstrator seemed young to me, childlike in her abashed pride in her art. Two of the pieces on display were made of stained glass and hung in floor-to-ceiling picture windows flanking Castelli's fireplace. One is filled with long, thin leaves or blades of grass in celadon, olive, and bright green. The leaves are apparently taller than a man or at least a child: they dwarf two human figures standing among them and peeking out at giant, luminous blue blossoms. The other piece shows more leaves surrounding a central column of purple circles like bubbles. A human figure, sexless and ageless like those in the other image, embraces the column. It would be hard for a work of art to be more about purity and the wonder of innocent discovery than these two seem to be. But after the Demonstrator showed them to me, she brought out a sketch for a painting she calls *The Scream*.

"It's pretty good, right?" the Demonstrator asked. What it was, was disturbing. "It's all these faces—that's all of me, right?" the Demonstrator said. "Most of them are not happy, right?"

"Here's a little Jesus up here," she said cheerfully, "and here's a little mouth and a tongue and an eye, and here's somebody almost dead here. And see the little fingertips touching the big fingertips, and the claws, hands turning into claws? I do that a lot. But I think that's a good one."

At this point I'm pretty sure Castelli switched to an older Judy.

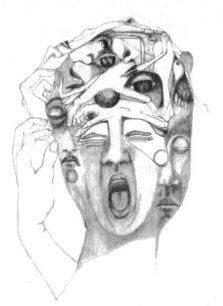

"Says something," she said, shaking her head at the picture, which she drew years before her diagnosis with DID. "God, that's what my brain looked like." Then she said, smiling, "Things are much quieter now."

Spiegel told me that for those with DID, mental health is reached by putting together the pieces of minds that seem as fragmented as the head in Castelli's picture. "One of my patients brought in a tube of Krazy Glue," he told me, "and said, 'That's what you're doing.'" And that is what he does, he says. "You try and glue 'em together."

Castelli believes she has been fairly successful at gluing herself together. Although in the beginning, "each part had their own history, they had their own life experience, they had their own memories, they had their own feelings and their way of behavior, based on what they lived through," Castelli said, "I am co-conscious at this point, which means I am aware of the other parts, and the other parts are aware of me, and we kind of share a consciousness now," to the extent that she can send information from one identity to another by conferring inside her head. "Sometimes I do have to say—I ask inside still, 'Is everybody OK? Is there somebody not OK with this?'" If she doesn't, she said, some of her parts may withhold information and then sabotage her work to make themselves heard. For example, she told me, "I was doing some piece of art, and I *kicked* it." She thought it was an accident, but, she said, "The next thing I knew I burned my finger on the soldering iron, and I thought, 'What the heck is going on?'" She couldn't figure out what the problem was, she told me, "until I said, 'What's happening?' and the answer came back, 'We're tired,'" and she realized it was time to stop work for the day. But aside from communication problems like that, Castelli believes she has reached a point in her life where she's satisfied with her mind the way it is. She is no longer in therapy, feels that her harmful parts have been integrated or relieved of their need to harm, and wants to focus on other things.

I asked Spiegel if he thinks that's a good idea, and he surprised me. "Yeah," he said. "They reach kind of what I call a metastable equilibrium. I'd say they're a little more vulnerable—if something bad happens—to get worse again, but, you know, if it doesn't itch don't scratch it." He told me about a male DID patient of his who was gay and had a partner. "They didn't have much money—they lived in this drab little apartment," he said, "but they had a very interesting set of relationships and sex lives, because his partner had, like, twelve different partners, you know, so they never knew on a given night who he was gonna go out with. And they kind of enjoyed it." Because the two didn't have much else in their lives, he said, "I thought, 'Well, what the hell do I have to offer that's better?' And he wasn't all that symptomatic, and he wasn't suicidal, and so I just left it alone. I said, 'Fine, have fun,' you know. 'Here's my number. Call me if you've got a problem.' And I never got called, so—sometimes, but it depends."

CASTELLI TOLD ME that what bothers her the most about portrayals of DID in the media is that usually the last person they show in a segment about DID is one of the scoffers. "I wish they didn't always go back to the doubt people," she said. "I wish they didn't go back to the ones that don't believe in it." So I'll return first to Phyllis, who said, "She's definitely multiple, and I never doubted it," when I asked if since Castelli's diagnosis she'd ever found herself wondering whether it, like the diagnosis of schizophrenia, was wrong. "I see them, and they're all part of her," she said. "I mean, she could wake up in the middle of the night and she could be a child. She didn't see that I was up and then got up and start talking in a baby voice. I mean she would wake up from a sound sleep" as one of her child alters, Phyllis said. "So, no. Never doubted it."

And then I'll cut to Spiegel. "I think there's something about the sort of drama of the disorders and the malleability of beliefs that scares people," he said. "The idea that our identity could be so changeable, that we could forget aspects of our past and suddenly have them come back, that we could think we're one person and think we're something else—I think it frightens people a little." Hypnosis does, too, he said. "I can, in a few minutes, hypnotize someone and give them an instruction about their hand and they'll act on it and forget what the instruction was. And it scares people." We fear such things because, he said, "we like to think we're more, sort of, planful and in control of what's going on in our lives and our bodies than we are, and I think these disorders remind us that we're a little more vulnerable than we like to think. So I think that's part of it—it's recognition of human frailty."

INTERLUDE: Adulthood

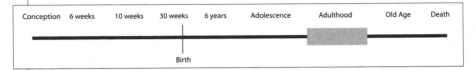

N ot much is known about the development of the human brain between postadolescence and old age. Most of us assume *something*
must happen between when we can't imagine having kids and when we
have grandchildren. But the truth is, the brain of a healthy twenty-five-
year-old looks a lot like the brain of a healthy sixty-five-year-old, at least
by the measures available at the moment.

It may be that the inevitable changes in personality and thinking as
we move through adult life are simply a function of our brains doing
what they developed to do: take in and store information. So it is worth
using this space to discuss how that happens. The following can be
skipped, but only at the peril (some would say) of failing to truly understand the enormity of the mystery confronting those studying the human
mind.

Today, if you were to pluck your cerebral hemispheres out of your skull
and somehow peel off the cortex and smooth out all the wrinkles, it
would cover an area about the size of an open *New York Times*. Within
that sheet of tissue, most of what we call thinking—the conscious planning and articulation of ideas—occurs. Long before the advent of laptop
computers or personal digital assistants or the iPod, humans carried
around the ability to compose ballads and symphonies, to not only learn
and use but devise the Pythagorean theorem, to remember birthdays, to
design bridges and evening gowns, to create and learn languages, to
find cures for maladies from rickets to ring-around-the-collar. As far as
we know, there is no other living creature, anywhere—and no nonliving
creature, either—that can do what we do with that sheet of neurons. But
how do those neurons communicate to form a new idea or a memory?

The answer begins with the neuron's cell membrane, which is made up of two layers of molecules put together to form a watertight film. That double-layered barrier also prevents most other molecules from passing through it—that is, from the inside of the cell to the outside. That impermeability allows the neuronal cell membrane to act like a capacitor.

The capacitors used in making an iPod, for instance, are basically two little metal plates with a bit of insulation sandwiched between them. When charged, one of the capacitor's plates has extra electrons in it, giving it a negative charge relative to the other. If the two plates in a charged capacitor are electrically joined (by a metal wire stuck through the insulation between them, for instance), the electrons from the negatively charged side will flow to the other side, discharging the capacitor.

In neurons, there is a difference in electrical charge between the inside and the outside of the cell, and the cell's membrane plays the same role as a capacitor's insulation, preventing negative charges inside the cell from leaking outside the cell and "discharging" it. In the case of the neuron, however, there is an added wrinkle: The electrons moving around are attached to charged molecules, or ions. The need for electrons also moves around, in the form of positively charged ions, to which electrons are attracted.

The two main players in a neuron's electric action are actually positively charged, meaning they're missing an electron. They are the potassium ion (K+) and the sodium ion (Na+). These ions float from place to place in the water that makes up most of our brains' mass. Inside a single neuron are roughly 15 billion sodium ions and 130 billion potassium ions. There are also enough negatively charged ions to electrically counterbalance those positive charges. The solution outside a neuron has about 140 billion sodium ions and 4 billion potassium ions. Negative ions outside the cell balance out their positive charges as well. Although the cell membrane itself is impermeable to any of these ions, there are tiny channels embedded in the membrane. These channels act like a wire joining the two plates of a capacitor by allowing ions (and their associated charges) to travel through them.

If the ions inside and outside a neuron were, like the electrons in a capacitor, only subject to electrical forces, those channels wouldn't make much difference: because the environments inside and outside the cell are essentially electrically neutral with respect to each other, there is no baseline electrical difference pulling the charged ions in or out of the cell. But an ion's movement across the channels, unlike an electron's movement along a wire, is subject to both electrical pull and diffusion.

The term *diffusion,* of course, refers to the fact that molecules tend to move from an area of high concentration to an area of low concentration. Because there is a much higher concentration of potassium ions inside a neuron than outside, potassium ions, if allowed, tend to diffuse out of the cell. Sodium ions, faced with the opposite situation, tend to diffuse into the cell. So because the channels in a cell membrane are specific to a particular ion (a potassium channel only lets potassium ions travel through it), potassium ions will use an open potassium channel to head for less crowded waters outside the cell.

As the potassium ions leave, however, they carry their positive charges with them. As a result, the inside of the cell becomes negatively charged with respect to the outside. Once that electrical difference gets to −94 millivolts (about a sixteenth of the difference between the positive and negative poles of an AA battery), the electrical force generated is enough to pull the potassium ions back into the cell, even against the concentration gradient.

When sodium channels are open, the same thing happens, but in reverse: sodium ions flow into the cell, since there are fewer of them inside the cell than outside. They bring their positive charges into the cell until the electrical difference across the membrane eventually becomes so strong that it begins pulling the sodium ions back out of the cell. In the case of sodium, that happens when the potential across the membrane reaches +60 millivolts, a positive value to denote that the inside of the cell is electrically positive with respect to the outside.

At any given time, a neuron will have some sodium and some potassium channels open, which means the resting membrane potential of a neuron is somewhere between that of sodium (+60 millivolts) and that of potassium (-94 millivolts), at −65 millivolts. When that potential is reached, the neuron is in equilibrium, with the number of ions leaving the cell balanced by the number coming in. Clearly, if left to continue swapping potassium ions for sodium ions, eventually there wouldn't be any concentration gradient across the membrane to keep up the electrical gradient. Maintaining the resting membrane potential depends on there being a lot more potassium ions inside the cell than outside, and a lot more sodium ions outside the cell than inside. So neuronal membranes have little pumps that use fuel from the food we eat to drive potassium ions back into the cell and sodium ions out of the cell, maintaining an equilibrium.

It is occasional fluctuations in that equilibrium, known as action potentials, that apparently allow our brains to collect, store, and synthesize information. Imagine a neuron in which there are about the same number of open sodium channels as open potassium channels. In many neurons, both the sodium and the potassium channels are voltage-gated, meaning they tend to open or close based on changes in the electrical difference across the membrane. In general, sodium channels are sensitive to changes that make the inside of the cell more positive with respect to the outside. For instance, if the difference across a small area of membrane changed from –65 millivolts to –60 millivolts, all the sodium channels in the region would open, allowing sodium ions to enter the cell.

That influx of positive charges would change the electrical difference across the membrane even further, perhaps from –60 millivolts to –55 millivolts, causing more sodium channels to open up and more sodium ions to flow in. If such a situation develops quickly, potassium ions can't escape fast enough to electrically counteract the onslaught of positive charges. In such cases, the charge inside the cell may swing from negative to positive relative to the charge outside the cell—from –65 millivolts to +40 millivolts, say.

But sodium channels tend to close once the difference across the membrane hits +40 millivolts. Potassium channels, however, are apparently programmed to open at just that point. Their opening allows potassium ions to leave the cell, taking their positive charges with them. Their departure returns the cell to –65 millivolts, at which point the newly opened potassium channels close and the cell is back at resting potential.

During an action potential, that opening and closing of channels happens sequentially along the length of a neuron's axon, like people doing the wave at a baseball game. And here is where the oligodendrocytes come in. When they wrapped their tentacles of myelin around neighboring neurons' axons, they only wrapped approximately one millimeter of axon at a time, leaving naked stretches of axon between the wrapped sections.

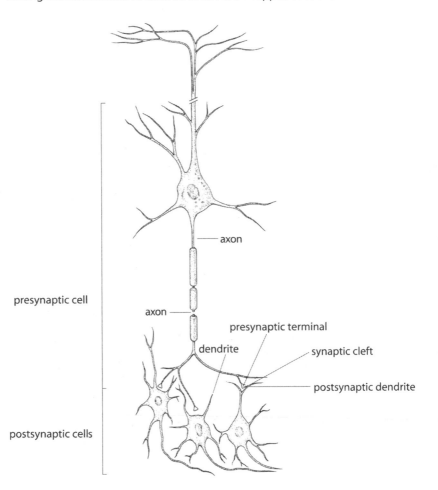

Those myelinated stretches allow an action potential to travel faster by providing electrical insulation. Picture two packed stadiums, one with wide aisles and one with no aisles. In each, the crowd is doing the wave. In the aisled stadium, the wave can leap across each aisle and so move faster than its counterpart in the aisleless stadium, where the wave must propagate for its entire course through the slow standing up and sitting down of people. The myelin sheaths provide the same type of shortcut for an action potential traveling down a neuronal axon.*

With the myelin's help, an action potential continues until it reaches the end of the axon, at which sit a collection of voltage-gated calcium channels that open with the change in electrical potential. There are a vanishingly small number of calcium (Ca^{2+}) ions inside a neuron, while in the space outside it there are approximately 2.5 billion, so that when the channels open, calcium ions come pouring in and react with calcium-sensitive proteins tethering vesicles of neurotransmitter at the axon terminus. That reaction allows the vesicles to fuse with the cell membrane, releasing the neurotransmitter into the synaptic cleft, where it can be picked up by the postsynaptic neuron. Depending on how much is released and what other signals are sent, the neurotransmitter may ignite an action potential in the postsynaptic cell.

The significance of the foregoing, and the reason to have waded through it at all, is that—as Francis Crick pointed out—as far as we can tell, every thought (wondering what you'll have for lunch or what you'll wear tomorrow), every desire (for glory, for that hottie you see at the gym, for a peanut-butter sandwich), and every experience (of reading this book, for instance—of your hand on the page, the quality of the light you are reading by, the feeling of your breathing) that you have or have ever had is nothing but the opening and closing of those ion channels and the release and uptake of those neurotransmitter molecules. One of the great philosophic questions forced upon us today is how that knowledge could or should change our concept of what it means to be human.

---

* We are completely dependent on oligodendrocytes and their myelin. In multiple sclerosis, a debilitating disease that can lead to numbness and paralysis, the immune system inexplicably and sporadically attacks the myelin sheaths and destroys them. Stripped of their insulation, neurons can no longer transmit the electrical signals required for a touch on the hand to result in a sensation, or for a desire in the brain to result in a movement of that hand.

*Philosophers think they can solve it by abstract thought and by using
a lot of words, and all the evidence of history is against them.*

—FRANCIS CRICK, on consciousness

*They're good at asking questions; they're usually very bad at giving
answers.*

—CHRISTOF KOCH, on philosophers

6 | Mind and Magic

Dr. Daniel Dennett, the philosopher of mind, is standing with
Christof Koch at the bar in Houston's, an upscale restaurant in Memphis, Tennessee. Dennett is holding a sweating glass of bourbon and
shouting to be heard over the happy-hour crowd as he continues a
long-standing debate with Koch over what has come to be known as
the Hard Problem.

Their argument predates the term, coined by the philosopher Dr.
David Chalmers in a 1995 paper titled "Facing Up to the Problem of
Consciousness." In it, he divided the puzzle of consciousness into
smaller problems in two categories, "easy" and "hard." What
Chalmers considers easy problems (and by "easy" he means they
could probably be figured out in a hundred years or so of hard work
by the entire neuroscience community) include more general versions of questions such as, How do you know the difference between
this book and a taxicab? How do you connect what a glowing electric stove burner looks like to your knowledge that it could burn you?
How do you know when you're miserable (or ecstatic), and how can
you tell someone about it? How do I keep plugging away, focused on
writing this sentence, while also aware that just at the corner of my

vision there is a movement that could be a hummingbird on my ter-
race? And how does either of us know we're not lying in a sleeping
bag beneath the stars on the Serengeti Plain, dreaming these questions while a hungry lion draws near? Those are, according to
Chalmers, the easy problems.

And the hard problems? There is really only one, in his opinion.
The Hard Problem, he said, is the problem of *experience,* of subjectivity, of the fact that I'm aware I'm me and know what that feels like,
and you're aware you're you and know what that feels like, and at any
given moment—even in our dreams—that awareness and knowledge remain, a backdrop to all the other conscious processes in our
minds. Understanding the nature of that phenomenon—or even developing a method to explore it—is the ultimate question for those
studying the mind. It is such a conundrum that it is inexplicable in
terms of anything else and thus calls for the invention of a new kind
of force or material, like mass or space-time. Or so says Chalmers.

At Houston's, where Dennett and Koch have come at the end of
the third day of the annual meeting of the Association for the Scientific Study of Consciousness, the two are rehashing their positions
on the subject. Koch is torn: as a practicing Catholic who raised his
kids in the church, and despite his rigorously scientific search for the
neural correlates of consciousness, he can't shake the feeling that
there might be something more than neural activity involved in consciousness, that our brains might only correlate with our consciousness rather than be the sole basis for it. Years before Chalmers wrote
his paper, Koch returned from a camping trip that he had been
forced to cut short when he developed an excruciating toothache.
The pain prompted him to write a letter to Dennett, whose work he
had read but whom he had never met. "To me," he tells me he wrote
regarding the pain, "there is this very *awfulness* that's above and beyond all the dispositions. For me in that context it's the most real
thing in the universe."

By using the term *dispositions* to mean behaviors and experiences to which we are prone by virtue of our physical makeup, Koch was claiming he had experienced a phenomenon defying explanation by the physiologic interactions of sense organs and the brain. He knew then, and knows now, that making this case was baiting Dennett. Since the beginning of his career, Dennett has unstintingly argued against the idea that anything we experience, including experience itself, exists above and beyond those dispositions.

"The key words there are 'above and beyond,'" Dennett says now. "It's possible that you're sort of doing double bookkeeping. You claim you're subtracting all of the dispositions and the effects, and you say, 'Let's subtract them all—and there's something left!' But in fact I think what you're doing is you're subtracting *most* of them, and the ones that are left is what's left. And then you're—have you heard my riff about 'The Tuned Deck'?"

Dennett is, more than any philosopher alive today, a showman. Along with his downy beard and the well-trimmed white fringe surrounding the smoothly bald crown of his head, the twinkle in his eye and air of magical jollity he radiates (even while puncturing illusions right and left) beg for comparison to Santa Claus. But there is also a certain hucksterish element to his charm. Dennett exudes the charisma of the barker in a traveling medicine show, and it's clear he's about to put on a spectacle.

"This is a true story," he says. "Many years ago there was a magician who was named Ralph—now why can't I remember? A famous magician from Ohio—Crooksville, Ohio."

The magician he's referring to is Ralph W. Hull, dead since 1943 but still well known among magic aficionados (of whom Dennett is one). It is typical of Dennett to try to credit him even in a barroom conversation. Hull specialized in card tricks and, in addition to hundreds of other ingenious feats of prestidigitation, as Dennett relates, performed one called "The Tuned Deck." "He did this trick for years for his fellow magicians," Dennett says. "Now. Let me put this down and show you."

DANIEL CLEMENT DENNETT was born in 1942, the son and grandson of men also named Daniel Clement Dennett, although the philosopher refuses to be known as Daniel Clement Dennett III. The first, his grandfather, was a doctor, an old-fashioned general practitioner in Winchester, Massachusetts, a town that even then served as a bedroom community for wealthy Bostonians. His son, Daniel Clement Dennett Jr., studied Islamic history at Harvard, then took a teaching job at Clark University in Worcester, Massachusetts. However, when the Second World War broke out, Dennett Jr. returned with his wife to Beirut, where they'd met when he was writing his PhD thesis and she was teaching English. This time, though, he was appointed the cultural attaché in the American Legation, an official title meant to hide the fact that he was a spy under the Office of Strategic Services, a job he continued even after the war ended. It was in 1947, the year his son turned five, that he embarked on a mission in a plane that crashed over Ethiopia.

After the death of her husband, young Dan Dennett's mother packed up the family, which included him and his two sisters, and returned to Winchester, where Dennett spent the rest of his childhood. Even in those days, he was interested in the big questions of meaning and consciousness. He remembers independently arriving at the concept of solipsism as a child (although this is apparently not unique, at least not among the philosophically inclined: he says about a third of his students at Tufts University, where he now teaches, recall having dreamed up the idea on their own). Unlike many philosophers, however, Dennett also had an early fascination with all things mechanical, to the extent that he says he would probably have become an engineer if anyone in his academically inclined family could have conceived of such an occupation.

Although he began high school in Winchester, Dennett spent his junior and senior years at Phillips Exeter Academy in New Hampshire, a place he calls "a wonderfully intense intellectual stew, where the editor of the literary magazine had more cachet than the captain of the football team, where boys read books that weren't on the assigned reading, where I learned to write (and write, and write, and write)."

That facility with language, along with his wide-ranging specificity—his work brims with references to subjects as diverse as Catherine the Great, James Joyce, Marcel Marceau, Milan Kundera, Casper the Friendly Ghost, masturbation, supercomputers, sailing, beer brewing, Tibetan prayer wheels, and the TV show *Candid Camera*—and his choice to write mainly in the vernacular, have given his work appeal outside academia. His 1991 book, *Consciousness Explained*, was chosen as one of the year's ten best books by the *New York Times*, and *Darwin's Dangerous Idea*, which came out in 1995, was a finalist for the Pulitzer Prize.

Dennett is also a popular speaker. A couple of years before I met him in Memphis, I attended a talk he gave at Stanford. The room reserved for him held four hundred but was so full when I arrived that I was forced to squeeze into one of the last rows. By the time Dennett took the podium, wearing a gray sport coat and the comfortable air of everybody's favorite professor, every seat—and every spot in which to lean, perch, or crouch—was filled.

In that talk, as in *Consciousness Explained*, Dennett continued an assault he began in 1969 on the "Cartesian Theater," a term by now so well known it is almost unnecessary to put it in what Dennett calls "scare quotes" (although usually only when they enclose words like *beliefs, desires,* or *choice*). Dennett named the Cartesian Theater after René Descartes, the seventeenth-century mathematician and philosopher of "cogito ergo sum" fame, who believed the pineal gland was the means by which our corporeal selves communicate with our minds. Although he recognized that we see through our eyes, hear through our ears, and use our brains to process information, Descartes believed the information then had to be sent through the pineal gland (which he called "the seat of the soul") to our minds, located somewhere outside our bodies, before we could experience it.

The pineal gland, nestled between the cerebral hemispheres, is one of the brain's only unpaired structures. It lies just above where the cerebellum and the brain stem meet, a bit higher up than the pituitary gland. If there was a separation between our brains and what Dennett likes to call "mindstuff," the pineal gland would be a logical choice for the communication between the two, and its function was long unknown. Today, however, we know that the pineal gland secretes melatonin, the hormone that may help regulate our internal clock and sleeping patterns. In addition, as my neurobiology textbook drily points out, the pineal gland's serving as the seat of the soul "now seems unlikely because pineal tumors do not cause the changes one would expect to find associated with distortion of the soul." So although how and whether melatonin regulates the sleep cycle is still being sorted out, and although it remains unclear whether melatonin plays the additional role of regulating sexual development in humans (as it does in other animals*), no one is very excited about the pineal gland any longer.†

That Descartes was wrong about the location of the "turnstile of consciousness," as Dennett calls it (employing a Dennettian rhetorical tool that might be called "refutation by ridiculous renaming" and

---

* A little-known fact is that if you keep male rats in the dark, their testes shrivel up— unless you've removed the rats' pineal glands, in which case they don't.

† Except first-year medical students. In our histology class, we had to learn to identify microscope slides of different organs by sight, and we all loved the pineal gland, which was easy to identify, as cross sections of it are scattered with calcified crystals that stain black in the slide preparation and are known as brain sand. That and the melatonin were the only things we were expected to know about the pineal gland.

seems merited in Descartes' case but a bit harsh when used to counter the work of living thinkers who are less obviously wrong), doesn't mean such a gate doesn't exist. Yet Descartes' view, known as dualism, is generally regarded by today's scholars as hogwash. At least officially. Dennett, however, believes a subtler form of the theory is alive and well and perniciously tenacious in much of the current work on the mind and consciousness.

This wrongheaded idea, Dennett says, is that information gathered from the outside world—or from the internal world of our own bodies—must be sent to some central place or "boss" in the brain in order to be experienced, that it must be displayed somewhere in the theater of the brain in order to be seen by the mind. He scoffingly lumps such beliefs under the moniker of the Cartesian Theater and insists that consciousness is not like a movie played on a screen or a play done for an audience. There is no audience, he says. If there were, you'd have to answer the question of how that audience, which Dennett generally characterizes as a homunculus, a little man inside your head, can be conscious of what it "sees."

It's certain that since well before Descartes' time, no scientists have believed there are little men inside our heads doing our thinking. But there are those who maintain it's reasonable to consider some parts of the brain to be unconsciously presenting information to other, conscious parts. In Koch and Crick's framework for consciousness research, for instance, they were clearly tweaking Dennett a bit when they suggested that the front of the brain could be usefully envisioned as a homunculus "looking at" the back of the brain.*

Such analogies are anathema to Dennett, who thinks that way dualism lies. As he writes in *Consciousness Explained,* that kind of

---

* Such tweaking travels in both directions: in print, Dennett has been known to pose arguments countering a hypothetical scientist named "Crock" who espouses beliefs parallel to, although actually far removed from, Crick's.

thinking "is not an innocuous shortcut; it's a bad habit"—one he believes gets in the way of our truly understanding consciousness. It's his contention that despite most scholars' outward rejection of dualism, it is so insidious and intuitive an idea, so tough to fully eradicate, that it continually crops up in the work of thinkers who would make (or have made) blanket disavowals of the notion. He calls such scholars "cryptodualists" and accuses them of simply pushing the problem of our minds' origin higher and higher up a ladder of denial. Much of Dennett's work involves chasing people up that ladder and, as he told me, "saying, 'And then what happens? And then what happens?'" If you keep going with that line of inquiry, he claims, eventually the pursued is forced to say something equivalent to "Ta-*daaah*—and the information is presented to the queen, and you're conscious!"

ON THE FIRST DAY of the Memphis conference, as I sat in the auditorium waiting for the first major talk to begin, I despaired of my ability to recognize Dennett amid the flock of portly, bearded attendees of a certain age. Nevertheless, when he arrived a few minutes after the lecture began, he was unmistakable: well over six feet tall, spectacles perched on his nose, the conference's free canvas tote bag an incongruous appendage. He chose a seat about halfway down the center aisle and pulled out a red bandanna to mop the crown of his head.

Many of my subsequent conversations with him were crammed into the time it took us to rush from lecture to lecture at the conference. As such, they were often interrupted by thinkers of various stripes accosting Dennett to talk over their work or simply say hello. They came from every level of the academic heirarchy, from award-winning tenured faculty to PhD candidates to the guy wearing a name tag that read "Independent Scholar" who cornered Dennett to discuss his own theory of consciousness, a graphic representation of which—in the form of a snarl of colored arrows and white text-filled boxes — he had printed on the back of his business card. One boy, probably about fourteen years old, nervously approached Dennett seeking an autograph.

That the scholars so eager to confer with him were neuroscientists and psychologists as well as philosophers is due to the fact that Dennett's work has brought empiric science and philosophy together to enrich both disciplines, and in many cases bridge their differences. During his career, although of course not solely because of his work, the line between philosophy and science has blurred. Dennett believes this is partly because in the field of neuroscience, "everybody really *wants* to be working on consciousness." Well, not everybody, he amended. "There are some neuroscientists — they're working on the brain, and it's as if they were working on the pancreas or the liver; they're interested in calcium channels or something, and they'd be interested in the analog in the liver. They don't care that it's the *mind* they're working on." But other than that misguided few, he said, "there's a sort of closet philosopher of mind in everyone in the field."

DENNETT'S OWN PHILOSOPHIC tendencies blossomed as an undergraduate. While at Exeter, he was interested in music and sculpture, but, he told me, "I decided I wasn't good enough as either a musician or an artist." Upon graduating, he went to Wesleyan University, where, ironically, he was introduced to formal philosophy when he read Descartes' *Meditations* and became fascinated with the problem of how a sentient mind can arise from the nonsentient materials of which we are made. It was at Wesleyan, too, while perusing the bookshelves in the math library, that he came across *From a Logical Point of View* by Willard Quine, a Harvard philosopher. He read it overnight, he told me, and was entranced by Quine's theories, although he came to the conclusion that "this Quine person was very, very interesting, but wrong. I couldn't yet say exactly how or why, but I was quite sure." So at nineteen years old, Dennett — about whom it has been said that he saves modesty for special occasions—decided he had to go to Harvard to meet Quine and, as he put it, "see what I could learn from him—and teach him!"

It was there that he met his wife, Susan: "Summer school in the summer of 1960. We were both taking a course on the history of the symphony, and we used to listen to the day's symphonies together—go to the library, get out the records, and listen to them and talk about them." She went with him when, after learning all he could from Quine, Dennett went on to graduate school at Oxford, where he studied under Gilbert Ryle, a hard-core antidualist who scoffed at what he called "the ghost in the machine," his term for what Dennett now derisively calls the queen, boss, or homunculus.

At Oxford, Dennett—perhaps primed to do so by Quine, a staunch empiricist—became frustrated with what he saw as his colleagues' willful blindness to the physiologic realities of the body housing the mind in which they were so interested. Early in his time there, which would have been around 1964, Dennett remembers a conversation with some fellow philosophy students about the nature of the phenomenon of a limb's falling asleep. "And I said, 'Well, you know, what happens in your brain? What happens in your nervous system?'" He says he was roundly laughed at for hauling in irrelevancies. "And I thought, 'Well, I'm sorry. I think this is important. I think you should know what's going on in the nervous system,'" he told me. "So I had a friend who was in medical school there, and I sat—I remember sitting down on the floor with this guy and getting out a pad of paper. I said, 'All right, tell me about the brain. What's it made of?' and he drew a diagram of a neuron. 'It's made of lots of these.'"

The minute he saw the picture, Dennett said, "I thought, 'Oh! You could hook those up in big networks, and by varying the connection strengths between them, you could have learning, if you had some sort of a reinforcement mechanism.' It just hit me—I just *saw* it, just like that."

Almost a century before Dennett's epiphany on the hallway floor, a Spanish doctor named Santiago Ramón y Cajal had come up with the same idea. Ramón y Cajal had wanted to be an artist but, at the behest of his father, became a doctor and a scientist. He is known today for his exquisite drawings of neurons. Although there is evidence that Ramón y Cajal theorized that learning and memory might result when a population of neurons reinforce the strength of their interconnections to form associative networks, he never formally proposed the idea, and it is usually credited to the Canadian psychologist Donald Hebb, who posited it in 1949, when testing it was becoming more feasible.*

Hebb's hypothesis has since been shown to hold true and has been succinctly restated as "Those that fire together, wire together." It says that neurons that are connected by synapses and that tend to be stimulated at the same time—say, a neuron in the fusiform gyrus that fires as part of the visual experience of your lover's face and a neuron that fires when you're happy—will strengthen their synaptic relationship. Over time, the theory goes, this strengthening means that when you see your lover's face as the lover's-face neuron fires, it becomes easier for that firing to result in the firing of the happy neuron as well.

Of course, that explanation is a gross oversimplification; most theories posit that more than one neuron is required for recognition of a face and certainly for love and happiness. But the point is that because of the strengthened connections between the two sets of neurons—one firing when you see your lover's face and one firing when

---

* Ramón y Cajal's work didn't go unnoticed, however. In 1906, he and the Italian pathologist Camillo Golgi won the Nobel Prize in Physiology or Medicine for their work on elucidating the cellular anatomy of the nervous system. It was the first time the prize was shared: Ramón y Cajal had used a stain developed by Golgi to clearly visualize neurons and study their architecture. Ironically, Golgi himself had been a proponent of the idea—already out of favor before his own stain was used to prove him wrong—that the brain was a syncytium, rather than composed of individual cells.

you are happy—the sight of your lover's face is (one hopes) more likely to induce happiness than rage, fear, sorrow, or thoughts of tax-law reform.

Hebb had already put forth his theory when Dennett arrived at it after seeing his first picture of a neuron, but the research indicating Hebb was on the right track had yet to be done, and at any rate, Dennett had never heard of Hebb. (Later, he told me, "I read Hebb and thought, 'OK, I can see other people are already onto this.'") Dennett's immediate conception of the possibilities inherent in the cellular makeup of our brains was both brilliant and prescient, requiring practical integration of information from science, philosophy, and engineering along with a healthy dose of intuition. As such, it was typical of him, as was the spontaneity and extracurricular nature of his first neurophysiology lesson. "I'm an autodidact," he told me, but then said, "No, I'm not. I've had wonderful informants and tutors over the years. So I'm not an autodidact, but"—like that first neuroscience tutorial—"it's all been informal." Also typical of Dennett was his reaction to that lesson. Sitting on the floor with his friend, a picture of a branching neuron in front of them, Dennett says he thought, "Well, I gotta know more about these."

THE EVENING OF the first day I spent with Dennett, we went to the Rum Boogie Café on Beale Street. It was a warm Tennessee night in late spring, and Dennett had had a craving for ribs and blues, now being satisfied by the Memphis Platter—ribs, fried catfish, beans and rice—and the Delta Cats, an unlikely but electric duo made up of a skinny white harmonica player barely out of his teens and a much older and fatter black man on guitar.

"A little confession," said Dennett, who did in fact spend the thirty-five years after he saw that first neuron learning more about the cells. "I find myself eagerly looking forward to a new psychology book, and not so much to a new philosophy book." Why? "Because with a new neuroscience book or something—even if the methods are bad, the thinking is wrong—when I get done, I've learned something. When I get done with a bad philosophy paper, I haven't learned anything; I've just learned another way someone's reasoning can be bad." These days, he thinks, "The really interesting philosophical questions occur right in the thick of the empirical work," which may be evidence of a passing of the torch that has happened before, in other arenas. "Philosophy is the mother," he said. "When you don't yet know the right questions to ask, you're doing philosophy. As soon as you pose the right questions, you can go off and try to answer them—and that's a new discipline: mathematics, physics, astronomy, biology."*

More evidence of the shift of philosophic questions into the scientific purview is provided by the group Dennett calls "the Nobel laureate carpetbaggers," men who began to study consciousness after winning Nobel Prizes in other fields. The group includes Francis Crick as well as Dr. Gerald Edelman—who won the 1972 Nobel Prize in Physiology or Medicine for his work on the immune system and now heads the neurobiology department at La Jolla's Scripps Research Institute—and Dr. Leon Cooper, whose study of superconductors won him the Nobel Prize in Physics in the same year, and who is now a professor of physics and neuroscience and the director of the Brain Science Program at Brown University, where he studies the cellular basis of learning and memory.

I asked Dennett why people like Edelman, Cooper, and Crick would be attracted to his field so late in their own careers. "I think in every case," he said, "the real reason is pretty much the same. They've knocked over one or two scientific problems, and then they look around and think, 'What's a *really* hard problem? What's Mount Everest?' and they come up with consciousness."

---

* Despite his enjoyment of the fruits of the field, "Psychology," he later wrote to me, "was born a bit prematurely perhaps, since there is still plenty of confusion about which are the right questions to try to answer."

The Delta Cats finished their set, and we stayed on to hear the next band, made up of seven guys—trumpet, drums, guitar, keyboard, two on sax, and a lead singer impersonating a seventies hepcat in a shiny polyester shirt and a beret, but who was nevertheless impossible not to take seriously. They played "Shake, Rattle and Roll." "Takes me back to my teenage years," Dennett said, and sang along with the chorus.

We drank more beer and listened to the music, and Dennett appeared to space out a little bit. I wondered what was happening in his mind, then realized his own theory could tell me. Sort of. In place of the Cartesian Theater, Dennett has proposed a model for consciousness and experience he calls Fame in the Brain. It's a theory that has its roots in the Hebbian synapse he intuited so long ago.

To illustrate it, let's say you are a philosopher having a beer in a crowded nightclub. The band is heating up; around you the patrons are clapping and stomping. The air is scented with barbecued pork and distant cigarettes, and occasionally the outer door to the club opens and closes and you feel the night air waft in. You are experiencing your life as an ongoing narrative: First you take a sip of beer and sit back in your chair, foot tapping. You begin to think about your upcoming talk at the conference you're attending. You make some mental notes, points you want to be sure you emphasize as you give what you've come to see as a retort to all who have misinterpreted or misrepresented your theories. In particular, you want to be sure you answer the multiple critics who claim you don't actually believe in consciousness at all. You have a flash of irritation at having to do such a thing, but then focus on the business of nailing down a logical argument.

A few minutes later, blinking, you look up and discover you're still in the club. You didn't hear the end of "Shake, Rattle and Roll," but the band has moved on to "Mustang Sally." You didn't notice when they started, but the people next to you are now dancing in the space between their table and yours. While you were mentally sparring, the mood in the room has changed dramatically, from pleasant and raucous to intense and delirious.

Did the music really stop and then start again the moment you looked up? Did the folks next to you silently and imperceptibly start rocking out? Did the vibe change at that instant? Probably not. Well, then, during your oblivion, were your ears unable to hear, your eyes deprived of the capacity to see? Of course not. Or absolutely, depending on your definitions of *hear, see,* and *feel.* Your ears were working fine; your eyes had the same capacity for peripheral vision that they'd always had. Your sensory organs must have sent messages to your brain. And yet you weren't conscious of those messages. So what happened? Did the messages get lost on the way to wherever it is that you become conscious of them? Were they destroyed? Were you conscious of them for a moment and then forgot?

This is where Dennett's Fame in the Brain comes in. There is evidence—much of it using techniques like fMRI—that in such situations the aural, visual, and tactile stimuli make it to your brain just fine, and make it to the same spots they reach when they're consciously experienced. So why aren't they experienced? According to Dennett, it's because they lost out in an ongoing battle with all the other things your brain has the capacity to be conscious of, including your breathing, sensations of hunger, memories of unpaid bills, the fact that children are dying in Iraq (and Somalia and Afghanistan and East Los Angeles), which underwear you're wearing, and so on. We have all had the experience of being ragingly thirsty, unable to think of anything but getting a drink until the moment we gulp it down, at which point we become aware of a ravenous hunger. Before our thirst was quenched, was our stomach not sending our brains the hormonal signals that make us feel hungry? Unlikely. We simply couldn't be conscious of them because the neurons responding to the hypothalamus's thirst signals (sent in response to increased blood concentration) wouldn't give up the spotlight.

In order to be experienced consciously, Dennett believes, a given stimulus (the drummer's solo, the cheers of the crowd) must not only excite some neurons in the brain, it must also excite *enough* of them to merit consciousness. How many that is depends to some extent on how many neurons other stimuli are able to excite. The brain, he says, is something like the reality show *Survivor*, with neurons auditioning in competition with one another to get on the island of consciousness, at which point they must forge and foster alliances to keep from being kicked off. While you're focused on your upcoming lecture, the neurons responding to the sound of the band team up with those sensing the people moving around you and with memories and other associations until they've got enough of a sphere of influence to earn the spotlight of consciousness. But at the same time, there are other alliances fighting for consciousness: the thirst and "sight of an empty beer glass" alliance is fighting for the idea of buying another beer; the sleepiness and "need to get up early tomorrow" alliance is fighting for the idea of calling it a night; and the pride and "desire to make a good argument and still be entertaining" alliance is fighting for continued focus on the upcoming lecture. Although no one knows exactly how much it is possible to be conscious of at once, we know that there is a limit, that we can't be conscious of everything at once, so Dennett believes some alliances get kicked off the consciousness island as others make their way on.

It's not always easy to tell exactly when an idea makes it or is ousted. Dennett gives the example of the phenomenon known as *phi.** Phi is what makes TV, movies, and flip-books possible. A series of still images flashed in succession, if they're similar but show slight

---

* To see the phenomenon, go to the Web content area of www.shannonmoffett.com.

differences in position, will give rise to the conscious perception that the images are moving. You can even be tricked into thinking that things change color, if the same image is flashed consecutively in different colors. So for example, if I ask you to look at a screen, and flash a red spot on it for an instant and then flash a green spot nearby, many will have the experience of seeing the same spot, first colored red in one location and then moving a short distance and, as it moves, turning green.*

The philosophic question this phenomenon raises is, How did you consciously experience the red turning to green? We know it didn't, but it felt as if it did. If we discard what Dennett calls the "extravagant hypothesis" that you somehow had a precognition that a green spot would appear, we have a problem. As he writes in *Consciousness Explained,* "The illusory content, *red-switching-to-green-in-midcourse,* cannot be created until after some identification of the second, green spot occurs in the brain. But if the second spot is already 'in conscious experience,' wouldn't it be too late to interpose the illusory content between the conscious experience of the red spot and the conscious experience of the green spot? How does the brain accomplish this sleight of hand?"

Seen through vision skewed by the scrim of the Cartesian Theater, Dennett says, this phenomenon would lead you forcibly to one of two conclusions, which he calls Orwellian and Stalinesque. In the Orwellian view, at some point you were conscious of the red spot alone and of the green spot alone. Once you'd been conscious of them both, a sort of mental Ministry of Truth rewrote history such that you felt you'd only been conscious of a red-turning-to-green spot. In the Stalinesque view, you were conscious of nothing until your brain had

---

* Dennett credits Max Wertheimer as the first to study phi systematically, in the early twentieth century, and Paul Kolers and Michael von Grunau for working with the color phi described here, in the mid-1970s.

gathered the information for both spots, then decided on an "official version," then displayed it for the masses, that is, the neurons that make up your conscious experience.

Both scenarios are distasteful, and not just because of the names Dennett's given them; we want to think we're conscious of things *as they happen.* The Stalinesque version, moreover, may be impossible: some experiments have shown there simply isn't enough time between display of the spots and subjects' responses to allow for all that processing. Yet that leaves only the mental rewrite team, which would still have to display its results to some kind of Cartesian audience.

But don't worry, says Dennett. We don't have to pick between those possibilities. In fact neither one is true, or both of them are. "The two theories," he argues, "tell exactly the same story except for where they place a mythical Great Divide." The difference between the ideas makes no difference, he thinks, because of the smearing of time and space to which our consciousness is subject.

To explain that counterintuitive idea, Dennett turns to evolution, which he became interested in via his study of consciousness and the brain. "The more I looked at evolution," he told me, "the more wonderful it came to seem. The people working in that field—well, (a) there were some really brilliant minds, and (b) they were philosophers." His fascination with evolution is such that it has turned him into something of an amateur naturalist.

Dennett spends his summers near Bar Harbor, Maine, on a farm he convinced his wife they should buy in 1969, although he was then still at the beginning of his career, an assistant professor at UC Irvine. ("I said, 'Consider the following argument: places in Maine are going to get more expensive faster than we're going to get richer, so we're never going to be able to afford more farm in Maine than we can now.'") The writer and computer scientist Douglas Hofstadter has called what Dennett does on his farm "tillosophy," but Dennett does sell hay ("when I can get a good price") and blueberries, and makes a naturally sparkling cider wine from the apples he grows there, picking and pressing the fruit in October and bottling the wine in May, both with the help of his students.

If he could, Dennett told me, "I would drop everything and study the beavers that live up near my farm in Maine," because "the beavers' dams are brilliantly designed, but the design isn't the beavers', it's evolution's." At some point in the course of the collection of random chance mutations that go by the name of evolution, enough genetic mutations arose in the mammalian line and were passed along to offspring that a new species was created: the beaver. But, Dennett pointed out, "you can't tell from any individual birth whether or not speciation has happened." Nobody can say exactly when the first beaver was born: At the time, had there been scientific observers tracking the birth of every mammal, it would have been impossible for them to know when the first beaver birth occurred, since they wouldn't have known which mutation was the last to develop. After enough time had passed—thousands of years at least—to decide that beavers were no longer changing significantly, the birth of the first mammal that would meet today's definition would have been lost in the mists of time. "You can't tell until generations and generations later," Dennett said, "which doesn't mean speciation doesn't exist, but that you can't identify it in this sort of straightforward, chunking way."

The same is true for consciousness, he says, which is why he likes to use the idea of fame as a metaphor for consciousness. We can say with great confidence, for instance, that either of the George Bushes is famous. And George Washington. And George Lucas. And George Jetson. George Eliot? Probably more people alive today have heard of George Foreman than George Eliot. But let's say Georges Foreman and Eliot also qualify. How about George Hincapie? He was a member, along with Lance Armstrong, of the U.S. Postal team for the Tour de France. Is he famous? Certainly among cycling enthusiasts he must be. He was almost a contestant on ABC's *The Bachelor;*

would he have been famous then? And then there is George Herbert, the seventeenth-century poet. Maybe he was once famous but isn't now. Well, when did his fame end?

Fame, if not a nebulous concept, is a category with unclear boundaries—much like consciousness, in Dennett's view. Just as it's impossible to tell exactly when the number of people recognizing a person exceeds or drops below the threshold of fame, Dennett believes it's hard to tell exactly when any element of what's happening in our brains gains or loses enough associated neurons to qualify as conscious.

Part of the reason it's difficult, he says, is that at any given moment there are a number of "drafts" of experience kicking around your brain, none of which can lay claim to being *the* official version of your conscious experience. According to Dennett, if we could somehow take a snapshot of your conscious experience at any given nanosecond, it would be different from one taken at the next nanosecond. It's only in memory that we finish the editing of our experience into any kind of coherent narrative, a narrative even then subject to change as we collect more experiences and thus more memories.

His subscription to that theory may explain why he believes in dissociative identity disorder, still called multiple personality disorder at the time he wrote *Consciousness Explained*. "The idea of MPD," he wrote there, "strikes many people as too outlandish and metaphysically bizarre to believe—a 'paranormal' phenomenon to discard along with ESP, close encounters of the third kind, and witches on broomsticks. I suspect that some of these people have made a simple arithmetical mistake: They have failed to notice that two or three or seventeen selves per body is really no more metaphysically extravagant than one self per body. One is bad enough!" But, he says, once you've allowed that one self can arise from the interactions of parts of a brain, there's no reason why—given some pressure to forgo the usually beneficial integration of information within our brains—more than one self couldn't reside there. He also points out that each of our brains could be said to have housed more than one self, albeit not at the same time. "Are you the very person whose kindergarten adventures you sketchily recall?" he asks. "Is (was) that child you?"

"The convictions that there *cannot* be quasi-selves or sort-of selves, and that, moreover there must be a whole number of selves associated with one body—and it better be the number one!—are not self-evident," he writes. That is, he says, they aren't obvious once you've gotten rid of the Cartesian Theater and with it the assumption that the concept of "self" is a central, undistributed property of brains. In Dennett's view, the word *self* is not a discrete noun like *rock,* but one more like *neurosurgical operation,* where the whole depends on the parts but not on all of them at the same time. Could Roberta Glick do an operation without a scrub nurse? Certainly, if necessary. Without an OR? Yeah, although it wouldn't be ideal (weren't ancient trephinations neurosurgeries?). Without a scheduler? Sure, though many have ceased to exist at the whim of one.

In the end an operation comes down to a surgeon and a patient, but even then, any surgeon will tell you there's always another patient; any hospital will tell you there's always another surgeon; and some scrub nurses have seen operations so many times they could probably do them. The quality of an operation may change as components are lost, and the nature of it may be altered by substitution of staff, tools, or location. But schedule a surgery for seven in the morning, then reschedule it for three in the afternoon, and then one by one change the surgeon, the scrub nurse, and the anesthesiologist and substitute another patient needing the same operation, and it's hard to figure out when one surgery ceased to be and another was created, if indeed that is the case.

IN THE RUM Boogie Café, the band struck up, and the singer yelled, "Mustang Sally!" to much cheering. Moments later, Dennett came back from wherever he was mentally. He clapped his hands and shouted, "Oh, yeah," and leaned in to me. "You must have seen that movie *The Commitments*?" When I confessed I hadn't, he said, "Oh, you have to see it. It's about this band in Dublin, and 'Mustang Sally' is their big hit." Could that have been the association that allied itself with the noise and the encroaching dancers to tip the song into his consciousness? Or maybe it was the saxophonist, now bumping and grinding with his instrument. Or the vocalist, who stood with his arms in the air, fingers pointing at the ceiling, calling forth the song? In any case, Dennett clapped his hands and sang, "Ride, Sally, ride," along with the entire crowd, which had gone wild. The singer pulled out a steering wheel from somewhere onstage, called up a woman from the frenzied audience, and put his arms around her, holding the wheel in front of her while she pushed the center of it as the keyboardist made a crescendoing horn noise and the drummer went crazy, and the entire place was drenched in chest-thumping noise.

We left after the song ended, the band tossing beaded necklaces to us on the way out. Dennett bought one of their CDs, and we stepped into the steamy late-night throng on Beale Street. Immediately outside the club's door was a spangly white horse and carriage. Next to it was a big red inflatable cocktail. "Good scene, isn't it?" Dennett said. "I think we struck it rich tonight."

In Dennett's theory, there are powerful influences determining the outcome for any particular alliance of neurons in its pursuit of consciousness. Some of these are external and beyond our control — the intensity of a band's performance, a nearby smoker — and some are at least partly under our own control. One of those is attention.

During the time I spent with Gabrieli, he told me about another demonstration by Daniel Simons, who did the "construction worker" change-blindness experiment. At the conference in Memphis, I saw the experiment firsthand, when the philosopher Dr. Ned Block used it in a talk. For the experiment, Simons had collected a gaggle of students, some dressed in white T-shirts and some in black. He videotaped them as they moved around in a space about the size of an elevator, passing a basketball back and forth among them. It was this videotape that Block showed us. Our task, he said, was to pay careful attention to the white-shirted players and to count the number of passes between the white-shirted players only.* Since the players milled about and the passing was rapid, this was not an easy task; but everyone gamely attempted it.

When the clip was over, Block played it again for us but this time told us not to worry about counting anything, just to watch the tape. Halfway through it the audience burst out laughing. A person in a gorilla suit had just wandered through the action on-screen, amid the T-shirted basketball passers. Almost no one had seen the gorilla the first time around, due to a phenomenon known as inattentional blindness. If you're not paying attention to something—even if it's enormous, unusual, and right in front of your face, and particularly if your attention is focused on something else—you simply won't see it.

This may seem unlikely: when I heard about the experiment, I was convinced that of course *I* would have seen the gorilla. I never got a chance to test that theory because, having been warned, I was on the lookout. But 50 percent of people don't notice the gorilla. The audience at the conference, accustomed to being shown holes in what we like to think is our unbroken awareness of the world in front of us, was still tricked. It's an eerie phenomenon, and it became even eerier when Block told us that, judging from fMRI evidence on similar phe-

---

* If you would like to try this yourself and you have a reasonably fast Internet connection, READ NO FURTHER, and go to the Web content area of www.shannon moffett.com. Once the video loads, press PLAY and carefully count all the passes from white-shirted players to white-shirted players. Then continue reading above.

nomena, the visual information about the gorilla makes it to at least some of the visual processing centers in your brain. In other words, your eyes, your retina, your optic nerves, and your occipital cortex all "see" the gorilla, but *you* don't.

Or at least, you don't know you do. Experiments like Gabrieli's and Simons's are now providing evidence for the blurriness of the border between conscious and not-conscious that Dennett proposes. (Although such a study hasn't been done, much cognitive-science research suggests that if you picked someone in the audience who hadn't experienced seeing the gorilla on the first run of Simons's video, then asked her a question like "If something weird were to happen in the next frame of the video, what might it be?" she might give an answer that included a gorilla. Perhaps she hadn't been conscious of the gorilla until you asked, but by casting about with the focus of attention, she might be able to elevate the image of a gorilla to consciousness, even without realizing where he came from.)

Dennett shows a similar (and to many, similarly unsettling) comfort with unclear boundaries in other aspects of consciousness research, such as the question of who is and isn't conscious. This attitude became clear at the end of the second day of the conference, when Dennett went to dinner with Block, who turned out to be the philosopher with whom Stickgold had argued over the fusiform gyrus's capacity for independent consciousness. Dennett regularly has similar—and similarly heated—arguments with Block (and has come to expect them: before joining him, Dennett patted his pockets and said absently, "What do I need? I should have a pen, in case I want to make a diagram or something").

When we arrived at the Rendezvous—recommended to Dennett for its barbecue—our table wasn't ready yet, so we sat at the bar to wait. The elderly bartender laid out cocktail napkins and asked, "So, where you guys from?"

"Massachusetts," Dennett answered.

"Hey, y'all, we got some Yankees in the haa-ouse," the bartender hollered, giving him a high five.

Once seated and served, Dennett and Block began talking about when and how consciousness arose in living creatures, a favorite topic of Dennett's. "Let's go to the simplest living systems and see how their needs are met," he said. "There's no need for consciousness yet, but there's already a kind of subjectivity, in that a creature makes a distinction between itself and the rest of the world: it protects itself and not the rest of the world. And we can get a long ways from there without having to invoke consciousness. We can get all the way to plants."

But, he pointed out, once creatures started to move around and interact with each other, creating more complicated problems for themselves and one another, Mother Nature ("otherwise known as the process of evolution by natural selection," as he has written) began to come up with more complicated solutions to give her offspring a leg up in the fight for survival. It is living creatures' need to anticipate threats that Dennett credits for the development of the capacity to sample the environment (which we now call sensing), the ability to try out different solutions (which we now call planning), and ultimately the "fancy intellectual talents" we humans possess. In his view, minds exist primarily to predict the future, helping the bodies attached to them to avoid destruction.

So when exactly did actual minds arise? Where along the evolutionary trajectory from plants to physicists did consciousness develop? Dennett refuses to hazard a guess. He believes that, just as an individual idea or percept can exist within our brains on a continuum from not-conscious to conscious, an individual creature exists on a continuum from not-conscious agent to conscious agent. Along that continuum, from the first replicating macromolecules in the primordial soup—for instance, the DNA molecule that (as he likes to put it) was your great-great-great-great- . . . grandmother—to ourselves, who are capable of composing sonnets, creating college-basketball pools, and programming computers to analyze statistics on the prevalence of gastric cancer, Dennett doesn't think there's a clear place where you can draw a line above which everything is conscious and below which everything isn't. "That, I think, is the same sort of bad question as, Is a virus alive?" he said when pressed on the issue. He often compares those seeking such answers—the existence of which would imply that consciousness is a binary state and thus can't be summed up by measures of brain function, which clearly exist along a continuum— to the long-ago scholars hunting for *élan vital.* "It's what the vitalists thought: 'Yeah, you got metabolism, you got reproduction, you got growth, you've got self-repair, but then there's the Hard Problem: What is life?'" But of course, he said, "when you've got metabolism, reproduction, self-repair, growth, you've got—that's what life *is.* There's not this extra thing that's life."

He predicts that, just as the question of what is and isn't alive fell by the wayside with the discovery of the mechanism by which something that isn't alive (DNA) creates things that are alive (us, gorillas, vampire bats, crawdads, hookworms, streptococci), so too will the question of what is and isn't conscious fall by the wayside when we understand how something that isn't conscious (proteins, perhaps neurons) can create something that is: us. But isn't it a problem, I asked him, to be trying to define (or explain) consciousness when you can't say who or what is and isn't conscious? No, he said, pointing out that biologists have never agreed on which creatures are or aren't alive, but are still satisfied that they share essentially the same definition of life. "The more you understand it, the more you realize you don't have to answer the question of whether or not something is conscious in order to define consciousness."*

---

* But, he said, it's important not to come up with a definition before we've understood all the elements that need to be encompassed in that definition, lest we suffer what he calls "the heartbreak of premature definition," an intellectual dysfunction he believes many of today's consciousness scholars suffer from.

Dennett doesn't even stop at living creatures when he considers what beings may or may not be conscious. He labels himself a functionalist, meaning he thinks neurons aren't necessary for consciousness and experience and believes any substrate with the right number and kind of dynamic associations could achieve consciousness—or at least some of the attributes of consciousness. And so, when Block asked derisively, over a plate of ribs and corn bread, "How about some robot," one able to differentiate between self and nonself, "—is it conscious?" Dennett answered with characteristic unconcern. "A little bit," he said, shrugging.

THE NEXT DAY, when I arrived at the conference a few minutes early for Dennett's talk, he was one of four men holding a cart bearing a desktop PC and lugging it down the stepped aisle of the auditorium, which was packed. Once everything was in place, Koch introduced Dennett and gave him the floor, whereupon Dennett put up a slide showing a block of text.

"This is a wonderful book by a friend of mine, Lee Siegel, called *Net of Magic*," Dennett began. "It's about street magic in India. He's an expert magician himself, and there's a passage in the book that has become a sort of motto for me. He says, '"I'm writing a book on magic," I explain, and I'm asked, "Real magic?" By "real magic" people mean miracles, thaumaturgical acts, supernatural powers. "No," I answer. "Conjuring tricks, not real magic."'"

Dennett then asked who in the audience believed in magic. No hands were raised, but Koch shouted out, "What magic?"

"Which magic!" Dennett pounced. "Real magic or conjuring tricks? If you say no, well, then I can say, 'Oh, come on, surely you've seen Penn and Teller and these other famous magicians. You don't deny the existence of those phenomena, do you?' Oh, yeah, but that's not real. Well, it's real and it's called magic. But of course it's not real magic. This semantic problem that Siegel draws our attention to has its counterpart in the study of consciousness."

He then told a story he hoped would answer critics who claim he doesn't believe in consciousness, an allegation arising from his refusal to consider that there might be more to consciousness than measurable, reportable results of brain function. The story was told to him by the philosopher Paul Churchland, who had invited James "the Amazing" Randi to speak at the University of Manitoba, in Winnipeg, where Churchland was teaching at the time. The Amazing Randi calls himself an "investigator and demystifier of paranormal and pseudo-scientific claims," and although he is a magician — in the sense that Penn and Teller are — he has made a name for himself debunking the claims of people like the famous psychic spoon bender Uri Geller, who maintain they have a God-given (or in Geller's case, alien-given) ability to break the laws of physics, rather than an aptitude for well-choreographed illusions. Randi performs many of the same tricks such "paranormalists" do, and he doesn't reveal their secrets, but he has notarized statements from other magicians confirming that they have seen his methods and found them to be naturalistic and mechanistic.

Which means the Amazing Randi is able to make his living off these "supernatural" tricks without claiming they are supernatural, but without giving anyone the satisfaction of seeing how they are accomplished. "So Randi gave his performance," said Dennett, "and then there's a question period. And one fellow absolutely stopped Randi in his tracks by arguing as follows: 'You claim to be able to explain Uri Geller's tricks, but you don't actually give us the explanation, and moreover, I think you're a real psychic just like he is. You have magical powers. You just don't want to admit it. And you see, the reason is there's only room in this world for one Uri Geller, and you're riding on his coattails by claiming *not* to be a psychic. It's the only way you can earn a living in this racket.'" The Amazing Randi, said Dennett, "found it very hard to prove you're not a psychic."

Similarly, Dennett said, "it's very hard to prove that counsciousness isn't magical. Because there's some people that are like that man. They're just so sure that consciousness is magical. If you don't agree with them—that consciousness is magical—they're sure you just aren't talking about consciousness. That's the problem that I'm facing."

He went on to ask the audience to imagine they were gathered for the purpose of studying magic scientifically. "We'd want to have a neutral method of gathering the data," he said. "We could do that. I mean, we could be a society, here, of people who had all sorts of different views about magic. Some people thought there was real magic, some people thought there wasn't, and the idea was to study it scientifically and find out whether it was real—whether there was real magic or whether it was all just conjuring tricks." If you wanted to do that, he pointed out, "you'd want to have a neutral, agreed-upon, objective way of gathering the data. You'd want to scrupulously itemize all the real phenomena and see how to explain them. That would be the problem. So in other words, among your data are not sawing the lady in half, but making people *believe* you're sawing the lady in half."

And so he came to "heterophenomenology." There are a number of consciousness theorists who argue that because thought (and therefore consciousness) is private, it can't be studied from the outside, or at least not in the way Dennett says it can. They say there are certain ineffable aspects of consciousness that therefore can't be studied simply by asking people about their experience, but that nevertheless exist and must be accounted for in any theory of consciousness. Some, like Chalmers, think a new kind of "stuff," or a new force, will have to be described and called "experience," and that we may have to describe this new irreducible universal from inside it. Dennett can list others, among them his old Harvard classmate Dr. Thomas Nagel—a philosopher who wrote the oft-referenced essay "What Is It Like to Be a Bat?" in which he argues that it is impossible for us to imagine another's experience and that it would be futile to attack the mind-body problem until we had completed the impossible task of creating a common vocabulary of experience with which to do so—and

Dr. John Searle, Dennett's academic archenemy, who argues that consciousness is a "unified field" and as such is not amenable to the kind of neuron-based research Dennett supports. Dennett accuses all of them of ascribing to "lone-wolf autophenomenology," of having painted themselves into a corner, since if what they say is true, there's no way to fully study consciousness.*

Dennett agrees that if there is something ineffable about consciousness, then we're stuck: we'll never be able to understand consciousness because we'll never be able to talk about it. But he doesn't think it's true, as he thinks each and every part making up the gestalt we call a conscious self will eventually be explicable.

AND THUS HIS USE of the tale of "The Tuned Deck" to make his point. In Houston's with Koch on the last night of the conference, after having given his talk, Dennett puts his glass on the lacquered bar and rolls up his sleeves. He begins miming Hull's card manipulations, swinging into a patter worthy of a boardwalk carny. "Boys, I've got a new *trick*, it's called 'The Tuned *Deck*.' I've got this deck of cards; it is *tuned* to the *vi*brations of your hands and your minds. When I listen: buzz-buzz, buzz-buzz." Dennett-as-Hull holds his make-believe deck of cards up to his ear, pretending to hear them buzzing. "Now, 'Buzz-buzz'—he's flipping through the cards, he's listening to the tuning—'buzz,-buzz, this is the tuned deck! Now, here, pick a card, any card.'" Dennett fans out his pretend cards and offers them to Koch. "And you pick a card," he prompts.

Koch picks a pretend card. "But don't show it to you?" he asks.

---

* At least one person I spoke to, familiar with and skeptical of Dennett's methods, rolled his eyes on learning the terms *heterophenomenology* and *lone-wolf auto-phenomenology*, saying, "Yeah, I'd like to talk about my theory, which is called 'supercoolmegaphenomenology,' and I'd like to contrast it with what everybody else is doing, what I'm calling 'knuckleheadology.'"

"You don't show it to me," Dennett says. Then, back in his cadence: "I buzz the deck again. I say, 'Now put the card back in the deck.'" Koch puts the imaginary card back in the imaginary deck. "You put the card back in the deck, more buzz-buzz, cut the deck, da-dah-di-di-dum-ba-bum, and I produce the card!"

There's a pause while Koch looks at Dennett blankly.

"That's it," Dennett says.

"But that's a terribly standard trick," Koch complains.

By doing so, he has, of course, played right into Dennett's hands. The fame of the "The Tuned Deck," he tells us, was not due to the trick's novelty, but rather to the fact that no magician was ever able to figure out how it was done. This failure was not for lack of trying, Dennett says, as the magicians took measures to rule out every trick they could think of. "And no matter what they did," Dennett says, "he could always do the trick. So they think that he's got something, some new wonderful thing he's got." Years went by, and still no one could figure out Hull's secret. But not long before Hull's death, Dennett says, "he wrote up his own account of the trick and he gave it to his friend" the magician John Hilliard, "who published it in, uh—"

"A magic journal," Koch, an academic to the core, offers.

"No, in his book," says Dennett. Published in 1938, the book was called *Greater Magic: A Practical Treatise on Modern Magic* and is one of the myriad on a seemingly endless variety of topics Dennett can claim to have read.

"And now I'm gonna tell you how the trick is done," he says. "Like a lot of great magic, it's simple. The trick's over before you think it's even begun. And in fact the trick in its entirety is in the name of the trick. And in fact it is in one of the words in the name of the trick. Which word?"

Koch and I hazard two wrong guesses, which leaves only—"*The. The,*" Dennett says, and he watches understanding dawn on Koch's face. "As you surmised, he's got the buzz-buzz, this phony baloney, he does an X-type trick. They think, 'That could be an X-type trick.' They prevent him from doing an X-type trick, he does a Y-type trick. They say, 'Could it be a Y-type trick?' They prevent him from doing that, he does a Z-type trick. And what he realized was they could only prevent him from doing one trick or another. He could always do something, so he just stayed one trick ahead of them."

Dennett is smiling now; he's on the home stretch. "And I quote him, God bless him. He says, 'The boys were all looking for something too hard.' And I say that's it! This is what Chalmers has done with the Hard Problem. He's said, 'Boys, I've got a new problem, it's called the Hard Problem,' and then he mesmerizes everybody into thinking there is this one problem, when in fact consciousness is a bag of tricks."

INTERLUDE: Old Age

Conception	6 weeks	10 weeks	30 weeks	6 years	Adolescence	Adulthood	Old Age	Death

Birth

The Central Intelligence Agency's *World Factbook* puts the life expectancy for women in the United States at just over 80 years. The value for men is slightly lower, at 74.6 years. Those numbers reflect a dramatic extension of our lives since the beginning of the twentieth century, when an American could expect to live about 50 years. That increase in life span means that what used to be an academic question—what happens to the human brain at 70, 80, 90, 100 years old?—is now a practical matter with widespread ramifications for our society. One of the obstacles to answering it is also a ray of hope for those of us who are or who love people entering old age: the answer differs depending on who you are.

Setting the specter of Alzheimer's disease aside for the moment, there is a normal decrease in cognitive ability as we age, beginning in the fourth decade of life and continuing at least into the eighth. But "normal" has been determined by the averaging of data from many subjects; that group decline can't be used to predict any one person's brain function as she ages. Some people in their sixties, seventies, and eighties will continue to score as well on tests of memory and cognition as subjects in their thirties. Others will suffer only a mild decline, and others—while still not meeting the criteria for Alzheimer's disease or other neurologic illness—will suffer a drastic reduction in mental abilities.

Recent research has shown that normal cognitive decline with age is due to deficits in one (or both) of two systems—executive function and declarative memory—rather than to a generalized decrease in brain function, as was previously thought. Executive function is mediated by the prefrontal cortex, the part of the brain just behind the forehead. (In fact, the evolution of the human prefrontal cortex—the largest of any animal's—likely forced the development of the outsize expanse of skull above our eyes that we call the forehead.) Probably the best way to define executive function is to describe what happens when it's lost. To that end, Phineas T. Gage is often used as an example.

Gage was a well-liked and respected foreman of a railroad construction crew working in Vermont in September 1848. One day he and his men were using gunpowder to clear some rock from their path. Gage was tamping the charge into a hole drilled in the rock, using a three-and-a-half-foot-long iron rod, when the gunpowder exploded. The explosion shot the rod—only about a quarter of an inch across at the end Gage was holding, but more than an inch in diameter at the other end—through his skull. Its point entered just under his left cheekbone, like a giant needle, with the rest of it following. The entire rod shot out the top of Gage's head just above his forehead and landed, according to reports at the time, some twenty-five yards behind him.

Gage was knocked down but wasn't killed; he may not even have lost consciousness. He did bleed a lot and later suffered an infection of the wound but was able to fight it off. Apparently the rod didn't damage Gage's primary motor cortex or premotor cortex, located just behind the prefrontal cortex. If it had, he would have been paralyzed. But Gage was up and around and physically healthy enough to return to work just a few months later.

Nevertheless, he couldn't do his job. Before his accident, Gage had been known as a careful, thoughtful, intelligent man, easy to get along with and good at planning a day's work and keeping his team on track. After the accident, though he could and did make plans, Gage couldn't follow through on them. Plus, he swore, couldn't get along with his co-workers, was stubborn yet mercurial, and seemed to have no regard for the consequences of his actions. Overall, he was "no longer Gage," as his friends and co-workers are reported to have said.

Later evidence from functional imaging and from other patients with damaged prefrontal cortices has corroborated what Gage's plight suggested: The prefrontal cortex is responsible for the suppression of inappropriate urges and for the ability to stick to a plan of action, allowing us to be guided by long-term goals rather than immediate urges. The area is apparently also responsible for some elements of memory—for instance, "source memory," or the ability to recall where and how something was learned. In addition, it appears to provide our capacity to remember in what order things have happened or can be expected to happen, and to plan accordingly. For instance, someone with prefrontal-cortex damage might, when adding cream to coffee, stir before pouring in the cream. Finally, the prefrontal cortex appears to allow us to integrate and use remembered information.

Many of these functions can be shown to be lost or diminished with age—the elderly may be disinhibited or may find it difficult to remember where they learned something, even while recalling the information itself. It used to be thought that such deficits resulted from the death of neurons in widespread areas of the cerebral cortex, since some studies showed diffuse neuronal loss in the cerebral cortex as subjects aged. Lately, however, with improved counting methods better able to correct for variations in brain size, it has become clear that there simply isn't enough neuronal loss, either in the cerebral cortex at large or in the prefrontal cortex, to account for the steep decline in some people's executive function. In addition, when significant cell death is seen, the amount of neuronal loss doesn't correlate well with the degree of functional loss.

Connections between neurons can be lost without loss of the neurons themselves, however, and what does seem correlated with age-related decline in executive function is the reorganization and loss of synapses. Some of us, at least, appear to lose synapses and myelin from our prefrontal cortices and suffer changes in our prefrontal neurons' dendrites as we age. In monkeys, those changes appear to be linked to the loss of the mental capacities associated with the prefrontal cortex.

The other faculty we lose with age is declarative memory. Sometime after our fortieth birthdays, we may find ourselves having trouble remembering things that would have been easy for our younger selves to retain: where we put our car keys, a daughter's phone number, the doctor's instructions for a new medication. As with the loss of executive function, the culprit appears to be the loss of a certain type of synapse—

this time within the hippocampus, in an area where neurons from the entorhinal cortex synapse on hippocampal neurons. The entorhinal cortex appears to carry sensory information from the rest of the brain to the hippocampus, presumably for processing into memories. Although the information has already been experienced and understood (you *heard* your daughter tell you her phone number, and you knew what the numbers meant), the loss of some of those connections from the rest of your cortex to your hippocampus may mean that as you get older, the information simply doesn't get stored in your memory.

So the loss of synapses in old age is common and not necessarily devastating. In Alzheimer's disease, however, it is apparently the neurons themselves that suffer. In the early stages of the disease, a protein called tau, normally present in neurons, inexplicably adopts a shape incompatible with its function as part of the cell's infrastructure. The altered tau proteins then clump together in what are known as neurofibrillary tangles. The tangles build up inside the cells, disrupting their function. This change usually starts with the neurons of the hippocampus and entorhinal cortex.

At the same time, in the same regions (and also for unknown reasons), plaques made of a molecule called beta-amyloid protein collect outside and around the neurons. Although it is not entirely clear whether they are the cause or the effect of the processes leading to loss of neuronal function and mental capacity in Alzheimer's, these two findings—neurofibrillary tangles and beta-amyloid plaques—are the physical criteria required for a definitive diagnosis of the disease. As the illness progresses, they can be found in widespread cortical locations outside the hippocampus and entorhinal cortex. The spread of the tangles and plaques appears to mirror the clinical spread of the disease, which progresses from a disturbance in the laying down of memories to a widespread and devastating decline in mental abilities: loss of social inhibitions, abstract reasoning, language capacity, and eventually memories of events so far in the past that they must have been stored in the cortex, without requiring hippocampal retrieval. It remains a mystery why the plaques and tangles in Alzheimer's disease begin to collect, and why they begin in the medial temporal lobe but spread so inexorably to the rest of the cortex.

Today, a diagnosis of Alzheimer's disease is usually made based on signs and symptoms alone. Without reliable tests for most types of the illness, the only way to conclusively differentiate it from other ailments that cause similar dementias is by postmortem examination of the brain for tangles and plaques. In the beginning of the illness, of course, there is no way to differentiate it from the milder decline in memory that benignly accompanies some of us into old age. That may change as we develop better diagnostic methods; already researchers are seeking ways to diagnose Alzheimer's early using fMRI. That search raises serious ethical questions, though. Is it helpful to diagnose a disease for which we have no good treatment? Would even one false positive be acceptable? Who should get such a test?

What do you do *with it, now that you know it?*

—JUDY CASTELLI

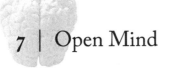

7 | Open Mind

ON A CLEAR DAY in May, 150 people gathered in an airy room at San Francisco's Golden Gate Club in the Presidio National Park. The hall's white-painted beams support a roof lofty enough to allow for a bank of twenty-foot-high windows. The windows look out over the sparkling bay, and it is possible to watch the progress of barges and sailboats across them, but most in the room had eyes only for what was going on inside it. A celebratory buzz arose from the group, making the occasion sound more like a birthday party or wedding than the academic meeting it was. In some ways, though, it was both wedding and birthday, as the event, a two-day conference called "Neuroethics: Mapping the Field," marked the official birth of a new area of scholarly research, as well as the marriage of the disciplines engendering it.

William Safire, the pundit and *New York Times* columnist, kicked off the event in his role as chair of the Dana Foundation, the private neuroscience-focused philanthropic organization sponsoring the event. It was Safire who had coined the term *neuroethics,* and in his talk he defined the pursuit, calling it "the examination of what is right and wrong, good and bad, about the treatment of, perfection of, or unwelcome invasion of and worrisome manipulation of the human brain." He also laid out the questions he hoped scholars in the new field would take on as their purview, such as whether science could or should develop drugs that might serve as "Botox for the brain," making people "less shy, or more honest, or more intellectually attractive, with a nice sense of humor," and what the ramifications would be if it did, or whether courtroom imaging of suspects' brains might be considered a way of forcing people to incriminate themselves and thus a violation of the Fifth Amendment.

Later, the neurologist and best-selling author Antonio Damasio spoke. His books—*Descartes' Error* and *The Feeling of What Happens*, for instance—have, like Daniel Dennett's, spread complex ideas from neuroscience beyond the academic sphere. Damasio discussed ethics in general, citing evidence that animals can experience feelings like sympathy, shame, embarrassment, guilt, and "the form of social anger we call moral indignation," and said that therefore our concept of ethics may have its roots in emotions we share with animals. But as with consciousness, he said, we humans have a brand and complexity of ethics that differentiates it from other animals', and that arises from our particularly well-evolved brains. "The upshot is," he said, "that ethics is a wonderful by-product. We could not have it if we did not have a capacity to learn, if we did not have a capacity to recall, if we did not have a capacity to imagine, to reason, and create."

In addition to Safire and Damasio, the conference was attended by neuroscientists (John Gabrieli was one), lawyers, neurologists, bioethicists, psychiatrists, psychologists, philosophers, science-museum curators, and journalists. In fact, among the host of luminaries present, there was only one who called herself a neuroethicist: Dr. Judy Illes.

The birth of neuroethics also marked something of a rebirth for Illes. Until just months before the conference, she had been working in radiology, the field in which brain-imaging technologies like fMRI developed. But "I really wanted to reinvent myself," she told me later. "And I started thinking about imaging; I started thinking about ethics." By her own admission, she knew nothing about ethics, but she had watched the development and use of functional brain-imaging techniques with fascination. "We were doing things we had never been able to do before," she said. "We were asking questions we had never asked before." It seemed to her, she told me, "that things were getting sort of interesting in terms of moral and social concerns."

So after spending ten years as a research developer and booster in Stanford's Radiology Department—where she landed after getting a PhD in hearing and speech sciences and then spending more than a decade at what she calls "the brain shop," a private research firm that studied cognition using EEG—Illes, an expert at garnering money from government sources, applied for a grant herself to study the ethics of radiologic imaging in general and neuroimaging in particular. When she got the grant, she moved her desk to Stanford's Center for Biomedical Ethics, where her first task was to aid in planning the neuroethics conference, hosted by Stanford and the University of California at San Francisco.

In her relatively behind-the-scenes role, Illes was all but invisible at the event. Although Safire thanked her in his address, he, like most people there, had probably never seen her name other than on conference correspondence. Her move from radiology to bioethics had her starting a new career in a new academic field in her forties ("young forties," she points out), and if anyone in attendance had paid attention to the fact that in this new career she was styling herself a neuroethicist, they'd probably have thought it a risky gambit. Who knew whether this splinter off the block of bioethics—itself only carved out as its own field in 1970 when the biochemist Van Rensselaer Potter gave it its name*—would stand the test of time?

* Van Rensselaer Potter himself envisioned the field as more global and more ecologically based than what it has become, which is a field of thought primarily geared toward addressing the many societal ramifications of Francis Crick and James Watson's discovery, with a tiny corner carved out for clinical ethicists to help doctors, hospitals, patients, and their families make difficult medical decisions.

Was there really more need for neuroethics than for any other organ-based or technology-based field within ethics? Why shouldn't scholars interested in ethical questions arising from the study and imaging of the heart band together and call themselves cardioethicists? or people who study the ethics of clinical drug trials call themselves pharmacoethicists?

The answer to those questions, put forward in various ways by each speaker at the event, was that new experimental and brain-imaging techniques, along with the push to develop mind-enhancing drugs, raise enough speculation about who is qualified to do those experiments, interpret those images, or prescribe those drugs, and about how the information gleaned or therapies developed should be used, that a new field is merited. Still, despite the big-name thinkers the inaugural neuroethics conference had attracted, it felt at the time as if Illes had hitched her wagon to a star that might burn out as soon as the meeting ended.

Which explains the look of satisfaction on her face a year and a half later, when I visited her in her office, as she tossed a magazine across her desk toward me. "Did you see this?" she asked. "I thought that was very exciting." It was the latest *Scientific American,* a special issue devoted to the advances in neuroscience since 1990, the year that began the Decade of the Brain by proclamation of the first President Bush. Teasers on the cover, which featured a glowing pink brain superimposed over images of drug capsules and EEG tracings, read "Brain Stimulators," "Mind-Reading Machines," "The Quest for a Smart Pill," and—the one that had so pleased Illes—"Neuroethics." The article it alluded to was an editorial written by the staff of the magazine, mentioning the "Mapping the Field" conference and calling for the further development of neuroethics as a discipline.

Illes herself had been featured in the media lately, following the appearance of an article of hers in the journal *Radiology*—not traditionally a publication that excites attention from the mainstream media. Her article reported on a study she and a group of students and colleagues had done on self-referred body scanning, a phenomenon that had emerged toward the end of the 1990s with the creation of centers bearing names like AmeriScan, Vital Imaging, and Early Warning Healthcare Institute. The centers marketed themselves as places where people Illes used to call "the worried well" (but now describes as "the health-conscious well" to avoid what she sees as insulting implications of hypochondria) could, without a referral from a doctor, go to have any of a battery of imaging studies to look for the cancer or atherosclerosis they feared they might have.

Although some of the centers also took referrals from doctors, they existed outside the traditional health-care system, were generally for-profit entities, and were utterly unregulated by the FDA or any other governing body. When I met Illes, the centers had also gone almost unstudied: no one really knew who chose to pay for such scans, what kind of tests the centers offered, or whether and how they followed the people they'd scanned. Which is why Illes's paper was published in an academic journal and got so much notice in the popular press when it was basically a write-up of the results of a Google search.

For the study, Illes and her collaborators used a couple of Internet search engines to call up a list of centers offering self-referred scanning, then gathered and analyzed some basic data on those centers. They looked at where the centers were located (mostly in California, it turned out*), at what the communities near the centers were like (mostly white, well educated, and rich, presumably the target client pool for vendors hawking a service that cost about a thousand

---

* At a talk she gave at Berkeley, Illes showed a bar graph of the distribution of centers by state, and the graph itself drew a laugh. The bar for California, which had thirty such centers, was more than double the size of the next bar (New York's, with thirteen centers). The bars for the other eighteen states in which she found any centers at all were arrayed to the right of the California and New York bars like so much background noise.

bucks a pop), and at how and to whom the centers reported the results of the scans. (Only one of the eighty-eight centers Illes's group identified said they sent reports to clients' doctors.)

Illes's paper also discussed advertising by the centers, noting that, as with much direct-to-consumer advertising for medical services, it played on people's fear of certain illnesses. In one talk Illes gave that I attended, she showed a slide of an ad for AmeriScan. It depicted a family of four, apparently a father, a mother, and two adult children, arms around one another, walking along a sandy shoreline. The mother in the picture was represented only by a white outline, which managed all at once to invoke ghostliness, absence, and the spray-painted outlines of corpses at crime scenes. The ad's caption read, "One heart attack. 4 Lives destroyed." The message, as Illes pointed out, was clearly that "if they'd paid to have a scan, they'd still be alive to walk on the beach with their family."

Illes and her coauthors called for advertising and reporting guidelines for such centers and also raised questions about the ethics of allowing people with no medical reason to believe they're ill to subject themselves to radiation and the worry and expense incurred by false positives, with no legal limits on the number of times the scanning centers could profit from their doing so. While couched in the dry and conservative language of academic science, Illes's paper raised the specter of money-hungry medical hacks taking advantage of and endangering the type of people who watch prime-time health-news segments, and not surprisingly, as Illes said, "the media picked it up like gangbusters."

But what about neuroethics? I asked Illes. Where is the connection between self-referred body imaging and neuroethics? The centers she studied all but ignored the brain, occasionally tossing in a "free brain scan" with full-body imaging, but mainly focusing on marketing their purported ability to make early diagnoses of disease in the rest of the body. Nevertheless, Illes saw her study as neuroethics by proxy. In one corner of her office is a poster she, John Gabrieli—with whom she collaborates regularly—and my classmate Matt Kirschen (of the Lego-voxel analogy) presented at a conference. It's titled "New Crossroads: Neuroimaging and Neuroethics," and on it is a quotation from Kierkegaard, written in 1846:

> What a sensation stethoscopy caused! Soon we will have reached the point where every barber uses it; when he is shaving you, he will ask: "Would you care to be stethoscoped, sir?" Then someone else will invent an instrument for listening to the pulses of the brain. That will make a tremendous stir, until in fifty years' time every barber can do it. Then, when one has had a haircut and shave and been stethoscoped (for by now it will be quite common), the barber will ask, "Perhaps, sir, you would like me to listen to your brain-pulses?"

Illes thinks Kierkegaard's vision is almost upon us, and when I met her, she said she saw self-referred body scanning as a precursor to its realization. Not long after I arrived on the first day I spent with her, I followed Illes down the hall to a conference room, where she did an on-camera interview with Tech TV. The segment was entirely about self-referred body scanning. But after it was over, while the cameraman was getting a two-shot and footage of a copy of Illes's article, she and the reporter chatted. The reporter said he was looking forward to the day when he could just decide to take a look at how his brain was working. "I would bet my last dime," Illes told him, "that functional neuroimaging is going to be out in the marketplace in the next five to ten years, and you and I are going to be able to self-refer for a functional brain scan."

It is that eventuality, Illes told me, that inspired her to study self-referred body scanning. She hoped to use it as a model to identify issues that might eventually arise with the availability of self-referred functional neuroimaging. For instance, Illes asked, "How often should somebody go and have their body scanned? Should it be once every six months? Should it be once every five years, every two years? Annually?" No one knew how often would make sense, or even how often would be detrimental, she said. "There are no data, there's no discussion, there's no nothing. But there's nothing that prevents somebody from pursuing these scans frequently, other than cost." The same would be true, she imagines, with functional neuroimaging.

Radiation wouldn't be a risk with fMRI, which doesn't use it and has been shown to be remarkably safe (although there is always the question of what might happen on the far side of wherever scientists have pushed the envelope of exposure). But on a more behavioral level, Illes said, "We really don't have good understanding of how these scans might affect somebody's lifestyle." Let's say, she posited, that "rather than having a good lifestyle, somebody says, 'I'm going to go get scanned every six months, and not exercise, smoke cigarettes, and eat fatty food.' I mean, I love french fries personally, and so maybe if I can be scanned, I can eat as many french fries as I want. Because if I have an early screen, and the screen shows something bad, then I can stop eating french fries."

In the same way, once functional neuroimaging becomes available outside the laboratory, people might use it to track the detrimental effects of recreational drugs, for instance, or, she suggested, to test themselves and their children for psychiatric or neurologic disease. Such uses might not necessarily be bad, she admitted, but as in the case of some genetic tests available for untreatable illnesses, they raise the question of what people — either the patients/clients or those running the testing centers — might do with information from the scans.

That Illes saw a link between consumers' ability to get a whole-body scan at what she called a "doc in the box" and their future ability to "get a little brain scan to understand why they couldn't find their car keys that morning, or scan their son or daughter because school started and they'd just rather be at the pool than back in class, and now moms and dads are concerned that little Johnny or little Susie really needs to have some Ritalin" is testimony to Illes's farsightedness. Or, a cynic might say, to her capacity to grab headlines in the present while staking out her claim to an area of ethics research not quite ready for prime time.

She makes a convincing case that it will be, though, and sooner than we think. Everywhere she looks in the field of imaging, she sees the smoldering possibilities of ethical dilemmas, and she has an iron in just about every fire that could possibly ignite into an area of neuroethical research. For instance, she conducted a study of neuroimaging research labs that use MRI, in which she found that the number of supposedly healthy subjects with incidental brain findings requiring referral to a doctor is higher than expected (about 7 percent). That finding raises questions about how research labs, not staffed with physicians and therefore ill equipped either to notice such abnormalities or to refer patients into the health-care system, should handle such results.

Although the incidental abnormalities found were all structural, Illes thinks questions over how to deal with such results may help frame future debate over incidental findings in functional neuroimaging, which she imagines might be less clear cut and more intimate. "I think we are going to be able to measure the pictures of our personality phenotypes, of our reasoning phenotypes, of our sexual-orientation phenotypes," she said. "We are going to be able to have pictures of our brains, of our own individual brains, that reveal information about us that we've never been able to look at visually and to appreciate visually. And that information is not simple."

Other studies in which Illes is engaged focus on the implications of the emergence of MRI scanning of fetuses and newborns, which she worries might develop into the use of in utero and childhood functional images as screening methods for pregnancy termination or school placement. In addition, she's planning studies on ethics and addiction.

And there's more. The Tech TV reporter said he had just been in Dallas, where a group was researching depression using fMRI. They were trying to make a "dictionary" of brain-activation patterns in depressed patients, then charting how those patients responded to different antidepressants, with the laudable goal of matching patients with the right medications without the long series of trial-and-error drug and dosage manipulations currently required. They hadn't had much luck, though, because, the reporter said, "Apparently we're not at that point yet." But how close are we to that point? he asked.

"That's a really interesting question," Illes said. "It looks like I will be getting a big NIH grant, of which exactly that question is one-third, which is: Where are we in using functional neuroimaging for diagnosis of mental illness, and how will physicians respond to that new quantitative information that we didn't have before? How will they change their practice patterns, how will they change their treatment, and how will patients view their disorders differently? And how will they comply differently, given, now, that there is a color map of their brains on and off drugs, for example?"

The truth is, at the moment we're nowhere near using functional neuroimaging for diagnosing mental illness. Almost all functional-imaging studies today average their data over groups of people, because there is too much noise in an individual brain for any clear pattern to arise, which is why the Dallas group wouldn't have had much luck developing their dictionary. The push for clinical uses of fMRI is strong—Gabrieli's lab, remember, was working on finding a neural signature for attention deficit/hyperactivity disorder, and other researchers are hoping to find ways to use fMRI to diagnose and track psychiatric disorders like depression and schizophrenia, as well as neurodegenerative disorders like Alzheimer's and Parkinson's disease—but it remains to be seen whether fMRI can be used in such a way.

AFTER VISITING ILLES, I went back to the Lucas Center where I'd met Gary Glover to learn about fMRI, this time to serve as a healthy control for an experiment Matt Kirschen was working on. Wearing a sports bra as instructed (the hooks in a regular bra can get hot in the magnet), I followed Matt down to the bowels of the building, where he seated me in a dim room to fill out the screening questionnaire Glover had told me about. I confidently checked off "No" when it asked if I had ever worked in a machine shop, and denied having a prosthetic heart valve, but then was pulled up short when it asked me if I had any other metal in my body. "Um," I was forced to ask Matt, cursing myself for not having thought of this until now, "just hypothetically, would a copper IUD count?"

After a hurried call to his boss, during which I was entertained by mental images of the IUD's being sucked straight through my uterine and abdominal walls by the magnet, Matt assured me that no such cases had been documented. In fact, I later learned, two researchers at the Robert Wood Johnson Medical School, concerned about just such a mishap, had put an IUD in an MRI scanner and monitored it to see if it moved or got hot. It didn't. (Although their experiment was motivated by case reports of women feeling their IUDs heating up while they underwent MRIs, the scholars' results were unsurprising, as copper is not magnetic.)

Once cleared, and after a practice session on a computer to get me used to the task I'd have to perform in the MRI, I was led into the scanner room. I lay down on the scanner's platform, scarcely wider than my body. The platform slowly receded into the white tunnel of the scanner, as if I were being slid headfirst into an igloo. While I lay there, Kirschen asked me to do the mental task he'd had me practice on the computer. It involved remembering a sequence of letters flashed on a screen in front of me. A few seconds after they were flashed, another letter would appear, and I was to press "Yes" or "No" on a little control box to indicate whether the letter had been part of the original sequence. Then he made the task harder: in the few seconds between the first series of letters and the single letter, a percent sign and a plus sign flashed intermittently on the screen. Every time the plus sign flashed, I was supposed to hit the "Yes" button, and every time the percent sign flashed, I was supposed to hit the "No" button, while still trying to remember the entire sequence of letters originally flashed, which could be as long as six letters. Then when the single letter was flashed, I was again supposed to push "Yes" or "No" to indicate whether it had been one of the original series of letters.

Kirschen planned to average my brain activation on the first task with all the other healthy controls' brain activations on the first task, average all our brain activations on the second task, and look at the difference between the two averages. Then he was going to have a bunch of people who'd recently had concussions do the two tasks, compare their two averages, and compare the difference between the concussion sufferers' two averages to the difference between the healthy people's two averages.

After the scan, I asked him if I could have a copy of my unaveraged scan. He looked at me doubtfully. "Single-subject functional scans look like crap," he said. And they do. When he showed it to me, there were colored splotches representing activation scattered all over the image of my brain. When he showed me the scan depicting my data averaged with that of the other subjects, all but two or three of the activation areas had disappeared. That average is projected on something called a standardized brain, which is itself an average or amalgam of a number of healthy adult brains, Kirschen told me. All the extra splotches on my individual scan show things *my* brain did during the experiment—thinking, "Oh, my God, I wonder if I'm the worst person at this task in the whole study," wondering what my feet looked like from the control room, feeling relief that a copper projectile hadn't shot out of my belly. Theoretically the splotches representing those thoughts and unconscious processes specific to me all faded out when the data from my scan was averaged with other subjects'. What was left, Kirschen hoped, was the common denominator, the areas of the brain used for the task he'd set us.

Even to say Kirschen averaged the data is an oversimplification.

The raw data pulled from an fMRI scanner consists of strings of numbers representing relative levels of magnetism in each of those one-cubic-millimeter voxels in the brain. And in fact, Kirschen told me, most researchers don't see those numbers; they see only the output from an initial program that does a lot of number crunching most cognitive neuroscientists can't tell you anything about. The data from that initial program are then analyzed using one of about four commercially available software packages for statistical analysis of fMRI data. Within each of those programs, there are a variety of ways to tweak the results using different analytical methods.

All this manipulation of the data calls into question the accuracy of the conclusions made from any given fMRI study, even one with a large number of subjects. "One of the things I'm trying to learn more about is how the black boxes of these statistical packages actually work," Kirschen told me when my scan was over. "I'm worried that using some of these parameters, you can raise a voxel above a threshold when really it's not." By varying those parameters, he said, "we can make activation centers grow or shrink, move left or move right— which is a problem." For instance, he said, let's say a surgeon preparing to remove a brain tumor is trying to map out her patient's language centers so she can avoid them during the operation. The surgeon would choose to leave in place any voxel interpreted as being part of her patient's language center. But any false positive, any voxel interpreted as being part of the language center when it really isn't, puts the patient at risk, since it could harbor a bit of tumor. Of course, false negatives would also be a problem. Voxels actually within the language center that are misinterpreted as not being part of it might be removed in hopes of getting all the tumor out, leaving the patient tumor free but with impaired speech, reading, or writing.

Such differences based on analytic method would affect the validity of results from fMRI studies of cognition. As Illes explained to me, it may be possible to take the data from a series of scans, "and if you manipulate it this way, you get a brain-activation pattern that looks like it's emotion," whereas "if you can remanipulate it this way, you get a brain activation that looks like planning." And, she said, "these statistical manipulations are all equally legitimate. I know that from back in my EEG days, where we used to do statistical corrections. We had so much faith that you could justify almost any statistical manipulation. You could. You'd go, 'That really didn't work out, did it? So maybe this correction would be better.' And in fact, we could justify this correction by the number of subjects or the number of electrodes or the number of tasks, pull out another pattern, and end up published six months later. So, was it the right statistic? Well, from many points of view, absolutely, because it could be rationalized scientifically. Is that a good way to do science? Well, probably not. But when you have so much data and you have such technological complexity," she said, "there's not really one right way." Trying to sort out that complexity, she and Kirschen have begun yet another study, comparing results of various statistical manipulations on the same data set. That such studies have yet to be done, even while fMRI studies on every aspect of mental function are being published in major academic journals and covered in the popular press, is one of the reasons Illes believes the field of neuroethics is not ahead of its time but in fact has catching up to do.

AT THE FIRST neuroethics conference, most agreed with Illes that functional neuroimaging is already on the path from prohibitively expensive experimental technique to boutique service for the health conscious or simply curious. Some went further. Arthur Caplan, the director of the Center for Bioethics at the University of Pennsylvania, said he foresees a down-market fMRI with a daytime-TV future. "I'll make a prediction," he said, "that in ten years there will be a show called *My Brain Made Me Do It*. Someone will lie in a CT scanner that quickly takes a picture of his head while the host asks, 'Guilty or not guilty?' Then, head image in hand, a test expert will come out and say, 'You know, his amygdala is kind of big. I think he did it.' The audience will then hoot."

Illes offered another vision for functional neuroimaging's use in popular culture. "What are we going to see a few years down the road? In personal ads of the *San Francisco Chronicle:* 'Thirty-one-year-old female seeks forty-year-old male for adventure seeking, risk-taking activities. Right orbital prefrontal and left prefrontal activations preferred.'"* Why not? she asked. "All people will have to do is go to the self-referred neuroimaging shop inside Stanford Mall, or on the corner of El Camino or something, to acquire an activation image of their brain so they can submit it along with their photograph."

I later asked Illes if she wanted to prevent such a development. "No," she said, "but I would like maybe to ensure that the reckless, cavalier application or implementation of the technology is avoided." When I pointed out that many would consider using an fMRI scan to snag a date well within the definition of *cavalier,* if not of *reckless,* Illes asked, "What's the difference between that and using brain images to see if people prefer one laundry product over another?" And so we came to neuromarketing.

About a month after the "Mapping the Field" conference, BrightHouse, an Atlanta-based advertising consulting agency with what it calls a "consumer insights arm" known as the BrightHouse Neurostrategies Group (it has trademarked the term *Neurostrategies,* as well as the term *Ideation Corporation,* of which it claims to be the first), sent out a press release. The document announced BrightHouse's intentions to use neuroimaging "to Unlock the Consumer Mind." For years, "marketers have tried to understand why consumers make

* Because the prefrontal cortex, as Phineas Gage's accident made clear, allows us to plan and integrate information in a way that we might call "good judgment," the writer of such an ad would be making clear that while she wanted a coadventurer, she didn't want one that was a risk taker simply because of an inability to conceive of risk.

purchase decisions," the press release said. "Although marketers have tested ad campaigns and PR efforts through surveys and focus groups, they still have not uncovered the emotional drivers behind the decision." To do that, it went on, what BrightHouse calls its Thought Sciences team planned to use fMRI "to identify patterns of brain activity that reveal how a consumer is actually evaluating a product, object or advertisement."

BrightHouse has a hazy connection to Emory University in that the scanners used for its research are Emory's, and many of the people working at the company either came from or still work at Emory. As a for-profit company, however, it isn't actually a part of the university, and most of what exactly BrightHouse does is hopelessly obscured in marketingspeak both in the press release and on their Web site.

When I called them for clarification I reached Dr. Justine Meaux, who is a research scientist and market strategist for the company. She was chipper but sounded exasperated—like Illes, she had recently been answering a lot of phone calls from the media. "We're not using neuroimaging in any new way," she said. The experiments Bright-House is doing, she told me, are "designed to better understand how people think, how they feel, and how they make decisions" and are inspired by "a desire to understand the brain and how the brain motivates behavior," which, she pointed out, is true of research done by academic scholars like Gabrieli, Stickgold, and Koch.

In fact, there are academic researchers, unaffiliated with Bright-House or other neuromarketing groups, looking at what drives us to prefer one product over another. One example is Dr. P. Read Montague, who studies the brain-mind connection at Baylor College of Medicine in Texas. One summer, he and his teenage daughter, who was spending her vacation working with him in his lab, did a set of experiments that received attention from the press even before their results were published in the journal *Neuron*. The two had decided to do a version of the Pepsi Challenge, but with a new twist: their subjects performed the challenge in an fMRI scanner.

They found that, at least judging from their brain activity, people preferred Pepsi. When the Montagues squirted an unidentified soft drink into the mouths of their subjects, a dose of Pepsi was accompanied by significant activation in the ventral putamen, an area associated with high-value rewards in monkey studies, whereas shots of Coke were not associated with as much activity in that area. This finding was consistent with the well-known fact that Pepsi does better in blind taste tests.

Coke does better in the marketplace, however, and the Montagues may have found out why people buy more Coke even though they prefer the taste of Pepsi. Or at least they found a clue. Because when they repeated the experiment but told the subjects which soft drink they were tasting, the Coke-associated brain activity showed additional activation in the medial prefrontal cortex, one of those higher-function areas that we believe integrate information but don't know much about. (People with prefrontal cortical damage, like Phineas Gage, tend to have abnormal emotional responses often described as shallow.) The activation pattern in subjects who knew they were tasting Coke may be evidence that it is our prefrontal cortices that take into account whatever the marketing wizards at Coca-Cola have told us to make us believe we prefer something we don't. Or, put another way, to make the net experience of drinking Coke, which includes all the associations those marketers have given us—the red can, candlelit renditions of "I'd Like to Buy the World a Coke," white polar bears and clean-cut all-American athletes—more pleasurable than the net experience of drinking Pepsi, with all of its associations: Michael Jackson's freaky-fakey hair catching fire, gyrating teenybop rockers like Britney Spears and Pink, and so on.

While Montague is a university scholar, with no funding from

Coke or Pepsi, it's clear that big corporations, for whom the cost of an fMRI study would be a drop in the bucket of their advertising budgets, are going to be performing just such studies. Or at least, clear to me. When I brought up Montague's experiment to Meaux, she said perkily, "That kind of research just goes to show the importance of branding." But when I asked her if the folks at BrightHouse were doing brand-specific studies like Montague's for their clients, she promptly answered no. Despite the fact that their funding comes only from clients—which include Coca-Cola, Pepperidge Farm, Home Depot, Kmart, Red Lobster, MetLife, and Delta—she said, "The big questions about how people think, how consumers think, don't have to be brand specific," and insisted that BrightHouse is simply doing "studies on preference, and trying to use neuroimaging to find a basis for preference," as well as to answer questions like "What is the role of emotion in decisions? What is reward? What is satisfaction?" They're doing "the same types of studies that other groups"—meaning other academic groups—"are doing," she said. "They'll be submitted to peer-reviewed journals."

Nevertheless, BrightHouse's use of fMRI has raised a few eyebrows, albeit primarily among the type of people who make the *Berkeley Daily Planet* habitual reading. Not long after I visited Illes, the *Planet* printed a list of "the ten worst corporations" of the year, compiled by *Multinational Monitor* magazine, a left-leaning monthly publication based in Washington, D.C. BrightHouse was on the list. And Ralph Nader's watchdog group *Commercial Alert* sent a letter to the federal Office for Human Research Protections asking them to look into BrightHouse's methods and their relationship to Emory, arguing that Emory was violating federal guidelines for human research by allowing their equipment to be used by corporations to "push products that are implicated in disease and human suffering and that impose great costs upon individuals, families and the society at large."

The OHRP found that Emory was acting in accordance with federal guidelines, but the birth of neuromarketing lends credence to Illes's belief that the need for neuroethicists is already upon us.

NEUROETHICS AND NEUROMARKETING are not the only new brain-centered subfields. There is also neuroeconomics, which although still a small discipline can count among its practitioners—or at least supporters—the economist Dr. Vernon Smith, who won the Bank of Sweden Prize in Economic Sciences in Memory of Alfred Nobel in 2002 for, as the committee put it, "having established laboratory experiments as a tool in empirical economic analysis, especially in the study of alternative market mechanisms." At first that work consisted simply of social experiments done with students in Smith's seminars, but today the field attempts to study human decision making using cognitive-neuroscience tools, like functional neuroimaging, and even physiologic tests—measuring blood levels of neuroactive hormones, for instance—with the ultimate goal of making better economic predictions.

At the moment, with functional neuroimaging providing only broad conclusions averaged over groups of people, the use of such scans in these new fields raises few worries about invasion of privacy. But as Illes points out, our capacity to use functional neuroimaging to make clinical diagnoses of individuals or reach conclusions about their personalities or past will likely continue to grow. If so, there may come a time when by participating in such studies, a subject could be opening the book of her own mind to researchers whose goals have more to do with profit than healing.

Once neuroimaging has advanced to the point that information can be gleaned about the state of an individual's mind, there are other potential uses for brain scanning that will certainly cause ethical dilemmas. At the "Mapping the Field" conference, Dr. Daniel

Schacter, a cognitive neuroscientist who uses fMRI to help understand what he calls "the seven sins of memory,"* gave a talk on what those sins and our new insights into them may mean for the future of human society. He told the story of a colleague of his, Dr. Donald Thomson, an Australian psychologist and memory expert, who had been accused of rape. The raped woman's detailed and accurate recollection of Thomson as her assailant led the police to him, Schacter said, but it turned out he had an airtight alibi. "He could not possibly have committed this rape because at the moment it occurred, he was giving a live television interview on, of all things, memory and memory distortion," Schacter said. "What had happened here was a classic though extreme case of memory misattribution." The victim, Schacter hypothesized, must have seen Thomson's face on the television just before or during the horror of her rape and had put the face together with the memory.

Schacter and others have shown that tricking memory by association in such a way is possible. In addition, once a misattribution has been coded into memory, Schacter may have found a method to differentiate between it and a true memory. In a study his lab performed, subjects were given lists that might include, for instance, the words *salt, sugar, sour,* and *candy.* After a brief study period, the lists were taken away and the subjects tested to see which words they recalled having seen on the list. Most of the subjects, Schacter's group found, remembered the word *sweet*'s having appeared on the list, despite the fact that it hadn't.

* Schacter's seven sins of memory include *transience* (the slow loss of access to a memory over time), *absent mindedness* (not thinking to grab your keys as you rush out the door until it swings shut behind you), *blocking* (which Schacter defines as "tip-of-the-tongue states and the like"), *misattribution* (thinking you read something in the *New York Times* when really you saw it on *Oprah*), *suggestibility* (implanted memories of the sort some people believe Judy Castelli's of child abuse to be), *bias* (where what you know now affects what you remember happening in the past: "I never loved that jerk"), and *persistence* (the inability to forget things you'd like to: "Why can't I just forget him?").

When subjects performed the memory task in an fMRI scanner, both types of memory—the true recall of items actually on the list and the false memories of items that weren't—were accompanied by activation in the hippocampus. The true memories, though, were also accompanied by activation in the parahippocampal gyrus, located just below the hippocampus. The parahippocampal gyrus didn't respond, or didn't respond as strongly, to the falsely remembered words.

Schacter listed a number of caveats when he reported his results, chief among them that they could be discerned only over a group of people—that is, the difference in parahippocampal activation in truly remembered words versus falsely remembered words is too small to be seen in an individual, only becoming apparent when results from many subjects are averaged. Nevertheless, if Schacter's test can be refined to show when an individual is experiencing a false memory, the development will have profound implications for our society and our justice system. The recent series of DNA-based exonerations, along with anecdotal evidence like the story of Schacter's wrongly accused colleague, raise serious doubts about the reliability of eyewitness testimony, even—or especially—when the witness was the victim. What would happen if Schacter's test could be used reproducibly and reliably in individuals, and if—a big if—it could be extended to cover memories of such complex events as a rape or a car crash or a witnessed murder?

Presumably there would be fewer false convictions. But would we feel comfortable putting every accuser into an fMRI scanner? As Illes says, "Fundamentally it could be considered an invasion of privacy, of time, an inconvenience—and who's going to pay the cost?" There are big questions just within this one tiny area of neuroethics: How much would change if we did have the capability to distinguish false memories from true ones? Would we find that the vast majority of eyewitness accounts are as wrong as Thomson's accuser's was? Would people like Judy Castelli, whose diagnosis and remembered past are cast into doubt, be exonerated or proved to be harboring false memories? What would we do about someone who believes with all her heart that her memory is true, even after seeing a scan showing it to be false? Would you believe a scan that told you the memory of your first kiss—or the model of your first car or the details of your last argument with your sweetheart—was false?

Functional neuroimaging is in fact already used in the courtroom, although not to verify the accuracy of witnesses' accounts. The scans are generally done with PET, which is cheaper than fMRI, and at the moment such images are usually used by the defense, with mixed results, in attempts to convince the jury that whatever wrongdoing the suspect is guilty of, it's due to brain malfunction. Such use may seem like Caplan's *My Brain Made Me Do It* come to life, but there's good evidence that some people's brains may in fact make them do bad things—or at least be incapable of preventing poor conduct even while understanding that such behavior is wrong. At the conference, Damasio invoked Phineas Gage and others with prefrontal cortical damage. Much study, he said, has demonstrated that the loss of executive function in such people doesn't mean they don't know how to behave well. "They know what is right and wrong and good and bad," he said, but they are unable to use that knowledge to suppress their impulses. That people with such deficits are as incapable of good behavior as those unable to distinguish right from wrong is a fact not well recognized by the U.S. justice system, but one many believe might be if there were well-established tests to diagnose them.

The possibility of developing such tests raises uncomfortable questions about the ability of any of us to control our behavior. Although Daniel Dennett and Francis Crick have celebrated the birth of molecular biology as the death knell of vitalism, those studying the issues that fall under the rubric of neuroethics remind us that with molecular biology came a raft of questions about genetic determinism, questions still unanswered today as the (some say misguided) search for genes for homosexuality, intelligence, and obesity continues.

Those questions have their counterparts in neuroethics, which one philosopher at the "Mapping the Field" conference lumped together under the heading "creeping neuroscientific determinism." He was alluding to the Specter of Creeping Exculpation, a phrase Dennett uses to describe what he thinks is the unfounded fear that learning more about how the brain gives rise to consciousness will make it impossible to hold a person—rather than her neural makeup—responsible for her actions. Later, Henry Greely, a law professor at Stanford who serves as the chair of an ethics subcommittee of the Human Genome Diversity Project as well as on the board of the California Advisory Committee on Human Cloning, discussed the difference between genetic determinism and neurodeterminism. Despite the hunt for various genes for sundry traits, we are clearly more than our genes, "given all the influences of environment, chance, and time on who I am and what I'm thinking about," Greely said. "The genes are an important part of me, but I can be certain that they are not my essence; they are not my soul." However, when thinking about neurons, he said, "I am not so confident. Is my consciousness—is my brain—me? I am tempted to think it is."

As, of course, we all are. Which makes it hard to decide what to do about evidence of brain injury or malfunction in criminals. What does it mean? Aren't all our deeds caused by our brains? Isn't criminal behavior itself a form of brain malfunction? (As Dennett has pointed out, this is a question that has been around at least since the time of Socrates.) What about neural plasticity, the recognized but still poorly understood ability of the human brain to re-organize so that a violin player can devote more of her somatosensory cortex to her fingers than the rest of us would, and a blind person can use her visual cortex to hear language? Couldn't the same be true of higher-level cognitive processes? If a criminal can be shown to have damaged her executive function areas — the areas that help keep most of us from following through on our uncivilized impulses — how do we know her brain hasn't adapted so that some other part can act to curb her maladaptive impulses? How do we know that despite having developed the capacity to control herself, she is nevertheless perversely and purposefully continuing her antisocial behavior? Should a brain that leads to criminal behavior and can be shown to have abnormalities be treated differently than an apparently normal brain that does so, even when we know how little we understand about the actual workings of the brain? How will we make use of our newfound capacity, crude as it is at the moment, to link the brain's activity with the mind's responsibility?

Neuroethics will likely have to tackle even more difficult issues arising from technologies beyond functional neuroimaging. In his talk, Greely mentioned Dr. Irving Weissman, a Stanford researcher intimately involved with California's stem-cell research movement. Weissman began his career studying immunology, eventually hoping to isolate human bone-marrow stem cells. Bone-marrow stem cells can become any of the types of cells our bone marrow is made of — red blood cells, white blood cells, and platelets. His lab eventually found the stem cells, and then went on to implant a human immune system in a mouse, allowing it to be manipulated and studied in vivo.

Now, Greely told us, Weissman is hoping to do something similar with neurons, implanting human neurons in a mouse's body in order to study them. Greely is helping to investigate the ethics of such an endeavor. "We have clearly realized that talking about a mouse with a human immune system — with human bone marrow — feels quite different from talking about one with human neurons," he said. "Because most of us would likely agree that the brain is somehow more involved in our humanness than is our bone marrow." That agreement, he said, shows that we generally subscribe to what he calls neuroessentialism. Although we may not believe the structure of our brains determines who we are and eliminates our ability to make choices, we do generally believe that our brains *are* us.

Suppose Koch ever does identify the neural correlates of consciousness and finds human neurons capable of experience even when disconnected from the rest of the brain. What would the neurons in Weissman's mouse feel like? If Koch does identify cells whose activation underlies experience, their discovery will surely have implications for, among other things, the tough decisions that have to be made for comatose patients. And who knows what Stickgold's work will reveal about the ethics of keeping people up all night in the name of military, medical, or commercial-trucking service? What happens if computers begin to show signs of consciousness, or if we eventually judge that Kanzi and Panbanisha or your dog or an embryo are conscious? Will they be given the rights we afford other sentient creatures?

Illes doesn't have the answers to those questions. Of course, right now she is focused only on neuroimaging. But even within that sphere, she sees her job more as that of question raiser than of answer provider. Every time I asked her about the ethics of any particular situation, she answered with another question. When BrightHouse opened its doors, Illes told me, a reporter called her to ask her opinion on the topic of neuromarketing and BrightHouse's new strategy to court advertising dollars. "And the fundamental question," she said, "was 'Is this an excessive use of technology?'" To which her answer, she said, was "Maybe." Later, she said to me, "Do I think we're going to be able to roll back the clock? Absolutely not. So should we wring our hands as a radiology community and say, 'Oh, this really shouldn't exist; we should stop it?' I think it's foolhardy to do that. What we need to do is move forward as a community in partnership, and say, 'OK, we're out there, people seem to be adopting this technology, they're hungry for more of it. Let's think about what we need now.'"

It remains to be seen, however, whether the neuroethics community will be able to keep pace with real-world developments. Just months after I spoke with Illes, I read in the news about the rapid decline of the entire self-referred body-scanning industry she'd been studying. It turned out there weren't as many people willing to pay the price as had been thought. But it may be that Illes was wrong about the centers' capacity to serve as predictive models of mainstream functional neuroimaging, yet right about the advancing tide of everyday neuroimaging. Just a few weeks later, I read an article about a psychiatrist who was "diagnosing" and treating his patients based on functional brain imaging— despite the lack of evidence for its use in individuals. The story said he charged three thousand dollars for a "clinical evaluation" that included a scan, and he had been so successful he'd established three more clinics in addition to his first, located in California. He had not published any of his patients' outcomes over fourteen years of alleged successful treatment but extolled the benefits of functional imaging as an essential tool for psychiatric evaluation and treatment. And in a statement Illes couldn't have improved on in her imaginary singles-scanning scene, the psychiatrist was quoted as saying, "If you date my daughter for more than four months, you have to get scanned."

INTERLUDE: Death

Conception	6 weeks	10 weeks	30 weeks	6 years	Adolescence	Adulthood	Old Age	Death

Birth

For most of human history, the failure of heart, lungs, and brain at the end of life were so tightly linked as to be indistinguishable. The easily measured loss of cardiac and pulmonary function definitively diagnosed death, and whether the brain's demise was the cause or effect of those two systems' failure was an academic question: if it hadn't come first, it inevitably followed. The invention of mechanical positive-pressure ventilation in the 1950s, however, meant that even without the brain's management, the lungs could be maintained artificially, keeping the body alive. (The heart itself, given adequate blood pressure—which can be maintained with drugs and the administration of fluids—often continues to beat even in the absence of significant brain function.)

The development of mechanical ventilation has had some extraordinarily beneficial results: we are now able to take over for the brain's most crucial basic function when it is temporarily incapacitated. Medical intervention can thus preserve a living body ready to support an injured brain when it recovers. In the frequent cases in which it fails to do so, however, this uncoupling of brain from body has forced us to rethink what we mean when we talk about death.

In 1968, in an attempt to keep pace with medicine's new abilities, an ad hoc committee at Harvard University set out to redefine the concept of death. The group comprised representatives from the medical, divinity, graduate, and law schools as well as the school of public health, and it is a testimony to Harvard's power and influence that it was successful in its mission.

It had become clear that the modern criterion for death should be irreversible and total loss of brain function, just as it had once been irreversible and total loss of heart function. The problem, of course, was that the brain is a much more complicated organ than the heart. The committee therefore set about making a list of commonsense criteria for the diagnosis of brain death: unreceptivity, unresponsivity, lack of movement or spontaneous breathing, lack of reflexes, and lack of electrical activity on EEG. They noted that if all those criteria were met, hypothermia and drugs causing central nervous depression should then be ruled out, to which end they recommended that tests for all the above capacities be repeated again after twenty-four hours, at which point a diagnosis of brain death could be made.

A refined version of the original Harvard criteria is now the generally accepted definition of brain death within the U.S. medical community. The most recent guidelines were published by the American Academy of Neurology in 1995 and require evidence of a cause of coma as well as the ability to rule out hypothermia, drugs, and metabolic imbalances. The original requirement that reflexes be absent has been clarified to refer specifically to brain-stem reflexes such as the pupillary light reflex (which causes your pupils to constrict in response to light) and does not include spinal reflexes such as the patellar tendon reflex, which causes your leg to extend when a tendon in your knee is tapped and may remain intact even in a body whose brain has been obliterated. An EEG is no longer considered necessary, although one is often performed, and the waiting period between the first and the recommended second evaluation has been shortened to six hours.

Of course, we all die of brain death, but in most cases the death of our bodies precedes the death of our brains. Whether our hearts, lungs, or other organs stop working first, the final common pathway to death is lack of oxygen to the brain. In a massive heart attack, the heart simply stops pumping, cutting off the brain's supply of oxygen. Within minutes, neurons will begin to die. Their death will result in inflammatory reactions such that, even if the person is resuscitated, the brain will begin to swell. If the initial damage was great enough, the brain may swell so much that it cuts off its own blood supply by compression, resulting in more dead neurons and more swelling. Obviously, death because of lung failure is similar: the blood can't get enough oxygen to carry to the brain. In the case of death from kidney or liver failure, toxins build up, irritating the brain, which eventually will swell, again cutting off its blood supply.

In instances where the brain is the cause of the body's problems, as happens with traumatic brain injury, the brain's swelling is the initial re-action. Enough brain swelling can incapacitate the brain-stem regions that regulate breathing, thereby reducing the drive to breathe. The logic be-hind putting patients on life support is that it can forestall such hypoxic brain damage if it hasn't already occurred and buy some time for the brain's swelling to subside if it has. If brain injury has already occurred, however, the damage is often irreversible, and one of the outcomes of our ability to keep people alive while their brains recover is that sometimes they heal just enough to no longer meet the criteria for brain death.

Perhaps part of the reason the Harvard guidelines were so easily accepted is that when they are met, the person usually *looks* dead. For most, in this country at least, it is easy to believe there is no more self held within the brain meeting those criteria. In addition, after a while on life support, the dead brain essentially disintegrates, liquefying and losing its structure, making it more difficult to imagine a functioning mind housed in it. So it is not brain death but the vegetative state that has caused most of the tragic battles over life support in the United States. A vegetative state occurs when severe brain damage spares some or all of the hypothalamus and brain stem. Thus, those in a veg-etative state can often breathe on their own. Their pupils react to light, and other brain-stem reflexes remain intact. They have normal sleep/wake cycles, but when awake they can't respond to instructions and don't make any meaningful movements. For the most part, they don't follow movement with their eyes or heads. They are incontinent of bowel and bladder and their swallowing and coughing reflexes, although intact, are insufficient for eating, so that patients in a vegetative state must be fed via tubes.

However, such patients may speak, though they only utter appar-ently random single words at a time. They may have "rage reactions," in which they scream, clench their teeth, and thrash. They may smile or moan; they may jerk as if startled. And every once in a while, a patient in a vegetative state recovers to some recognizable consciousness, although almost never after existing in such a state for more than a year.

It is impossible to know whether a patient in a vegetative state is experiencing anything when she screams or smiles. But of course, it is also impossible to know whether people who are brain dead have experience. When forced to, we've drawn a line at what we consider the most reasonable place between life and death. But the battles—political and personal, philosophic and financial—raging along that line reflect how much we don't know about the brain and its relation to consciousness.

8 | Mind and Body

I'M SITTING ON A ROUND black cushion atop a square black cushion atop a honey-colored hardwood floor in a simple rectangular room. I am staring at the wall. Around me are about thirty people similarly seated, also staring at the wall. One of those people is Norman Fischer, who, despite having been raised Jewish in Pittston, Pennsylvania, is a Zen monk. I met him just hours ago, in the Puerto Vallarta airport. He is fifty-six years old, and at the time, he was wearing olive chinos, a blue button-down shirt, an oatmeal sweater-vest, and Nikes. Nothing about him suggested he'd be more comfortable talking about what he says is his favorite subject, the thirteenth-century Japanese scholar Eihei Dogen, than about where to find a good game of golf. But now he is barefoot, a soft brown calf-length robe in place of the California casual wear. His hair suddenly looks more shaved than close cropped; his face, even behind silver wire-rimmed glasses, looks more chiseled than nebbishy; and he could no longer be mistaken for a tax attorney on holiday.

The *zendo* where we are seated is on the second floor of an ocean-front retreat center in Chacala, a tiny fishing village in Mexico still recovering from a recent hurricane. The wall in the zendo is white plaster. There is a mark in front of me, just below eye level, where the plasterer lifted the trowel. The mark is shaped like a fishhook. I will get to know this mark well. Months later I will be able to conjure it up in my mind, the way it looks lemon yellow at sunrise, pure white at noon, and at sunset when it is the color of a ripe persimmon.

We have been sitting in silence for maybe twenty minutes, the only sound the rumble-rush of the waves, when someone hits a little metal cup with a little wooden stick, making a clear chime, and Fischer begins to speak. He explains how things will work at this *sesshin,* a word taken from the Japanese *setsu* (to touch, to join) and the Chinese word *shin* (the mind, the heart) and usually translated as "to touch the mind" or "to collect the mind." In Zen practice it can also mean simply "a retreat," as a sesshin usually lasts several days and is set in a remote—and often beautiful—place. Those days are spent in meditation, chanting, and mindful work.

They are also spent in silence, with a strict ban on talking except during special sessions with the leader and teacher, in this case Fischer, who may also speak at other times. Now he tells us that we must not only take our shoes off before entering the zendo but also pay attention to how we put them on the shoe rack outside the door, and that we should be alert the moment we set foot inside that door. Which side of the door we should step to once inside is dictated by which side of the room we'll be sitting on, which is in turn dictated by a seating chart posted on the wall outside the zendo. After entering the room, we must bow, putting our two hands together, Fischer says, "to signify the two parts of our soul—the part that comes from conditioning, from how our parents raised us and society, and the part that is limitless, boundless." Then we are to walk slowly and mindfully to our spots, pull our cushions toward us, bow, turn around, bow, sit down, and turn around again to face the wall—eyes open, with our spines straight (but with a slight curve at the base), our chins tucked, our hands forming an oval at waist height as if we were cupping an egg in them—and begin meditating.

"These rules may seem stupid and annoying," Fischer says, echoing my thoughts exactly, "and they are. But it is to take you out of the stupid, annoying things that you are doing almost constantly in your daily life that we do them." A moment later he says, "What you are trying to do" — in *zazen,* the kind of meditation practiced by Soto Buddhists, the kind that involves sitting on the cushions, looking at the wall, cupping the imaginary egg, and trying to empty your mind of all thoughts but the feeling of breathing—"is to understand the experience of being a human being right now, at this moment."

Lovely. I've been interviewing people for months, people who've been working on only *facets* of that question for decades, and now we're supposed to find the answer in half an hour, while our hips are on fire and our backs seize up and the chorus of "(I Can't Get No) Satisfaction" by the Stones plays on an interminable loop in our heads. Oh, and by the way, "if your knees hurt or your back hurts, just breathe," Fischer offers. "Maybe you'll feel pain, or desperation. That's good. If we haven't explored deeply the way we are when we're in pain or desperate, we don't know ourselves very well."

Knowing oneself well is one of the goals of Zen practice, although it's also not a goal at all, because goal-lessness is another of the goals of Zen practice. In one of his books, *Turn Left in Order to Go Right* (a collection of poetry—he is also a poet with an MFA from the prestigious Iowa Writers' Workshop), Fischer writes that Zen is "not the usual kind of activity in that you can't really try to do it. If you try to move toward it it always seems to be somewhere else. The harder you try the worse it gets. But you can't not make any effort either; in fact you have to make a mighty effort, but in another direction." Thus the title of his book, and thus the difficulty, especially for Western minds—bred on rationalism, the scientific method, and the theory that the shortest path between two points is a straight line—in grasping Zen precepts.

Zen practice takes years, by all accounts, to even begin to understand (a word like Robert Heinlein's *grok* might be a better term for what one begins to do after practicing it seriously). A part of that process is learning not to think in absolutes. Like Dennett, Fischer and other Zen Buddhists train themselves and encourage the world to abandon dualist thinking. The term means something different to them than to Western thinkers, however. In the Zen tradition, dualism refers to the idea that there are two sides to any question, one of which is true and one of which is not-true. Such black-and-white divisions are not in keeping with the Zen worldview. (Dennett's pitched battle against dualism in the sense he means it—the idea that our minds are somehow separate from our brains—is a perfect example of the kind of dualism Buddhists try to guard against.) Fischer acknowledges, though, that to condemn dualism in the Zen sense is itself dualistic, "because it implies that non-dual is good and dualistic is bad. But dualistic is also part of non-dualistic. The real non-dualistic is both non-dualistic and dualistic."

This comfort in the absence of absolutes means that when studying Zen, it's important to understand that the words of any particular Zen teacher at any particular time may only be true at that time, in that context, and spoken to that audience. For instance, Fischer tells a story about Shunryu Suzuki. Suzuki, who died in 1971, was the first abbot of the San Francisco Zen Center, which he founded in 1962. (Fischer later served as its coabbot from 1995 to 2000.) Suzuki is generally credited with bringing Zen Buddhism to the European American population of the United States, both through his teaching and through a book called *Zen Mind, Beginner's Mind*, transcripts of talks he gave during his career. *Zen Mind* serves, along with other, older texts, as something like a bible for Fischer and other Zen Buddhists in the United States.

The story about Suzuki has it that one day, while he was on a long drive with a student, the two decided to stop for lunch. The student was what Fischer calls "an ardent vegetarian" and was exceedingly distressed at the apparent dearth of meatless offerings at the roadside eateries. Nevertheless they stopped, and the student ordered the time-honored choice of vegetarians in such places: a grilled cheese sandwich. It was to his great surprise that Suzuki, going against Buddhist teaching and his own long standing habit, ordered a hamburger. The student said nothing, not wanting to challenge his teacher. When the food came, as Fischer tells the story, Suzuki wordlessly pushed the hamburger toward his student, taking the grilled cheese for himself.

For most of his adult life, Fischer was also a vegetarian. But recently his wife, who is not, went on the Atkins diet. He decided to join her so that at last, after a quarter century of marriage, they could eat the same thing for dinner. He interprets the story about Suzuki and the vegetarian as showing that Suzuki "was trying to get the student to be less doctrinaire—not to be stuck on vegetarianism as righteousness, but to recognize that it's good to be vegetarian, but also, it's better to let go of all preconceptions and all ideologies and all firm convictions and have an open mind."*

The Buddhist tradition on which this ideology-of-no-ideologies is based began with the life and teachings of Siddhartha Gautama, born to an aristocratic family about twenty-five hundred years ago in what is now Nepal. Siddhartha was raised in a state of sheltered luxury after it was foretold to his father, Suddhodana, that Siddhartha would be either a great and powerful king or an enlightened religious leader. Preferring the former, Suddhodana tried to protect his son from the suffering of the world, exposure to which he felt would more likely induce him to take up religion.

Suddhodana's strategy worked longer than might have been expected. But one day when Siddhartha was twenty-nine, already

---

* Other people's versions of the story have Suzuki taking a bite of the hamburger, saying, "I don't like this. Here, you eat it," and handing it to his student, which allows for different interpretations and highlights the fallibility—acknowledged by both Eastern and Western thought—of human memory.

married and a father, he went for a ride in his chariot. On that outing, he saw an old man, hobbling and infirm. A bit farther along, he saw a sick man. After that, he came upon a group of mourners carrying a corpse to its funeral pyre. According to Buddhist tradition, that day was the first that Siddhartha had ever witnessed human pain and grief. Once he learned of their existence, he became obsessed with the desire to understand them, convinced that if he could grasp the nature of and reasons for suffering, he could thereby discover the path to their elimination.

In an attempt to experience and so comprehend such misery, Siddhartha left his comfortable life and his family. He met and followed a group of ascetics who practiced extreme austerity, eating next to nothing and depriving themselves of all physical pleasures. After six years with them, when he still had not attained understanding, Siddhartha stopped eating altogether and came close to starving. At last, when he was nearly dead, a peasant girl offered him some milk, which he took and drank, at which point he realized that his agony had not provided the clarity he sought. Undeterred from his mission, however, he changed tactics. He decided he would sit under a tree—a fig tree, as the story goes, now known as the bodhi, or "awakening," tree—until he understood.

There he sat for seven days and seven nights, until at last he achieved enlightenment and, now the Buddha (the Awakened), realized what are known in Buddhism as the four noble truths: that suffering is universal, that ignorance is the source of suffering, that suffering can be overcome, and that the way to overcome it is the eightfold path. The eightfold path involves practicing right view, right intention, right speech, right action, right livelihood, right effort, right mindfulness, and right concentration. Buddhists today try to live by those tenets and, when they meditate, are following Siddhartha's example, attempting to open themselves to enlightenment by sitting still as he did under the bodhi tree.

So in the zendo, after Fischer's instructions, the little stick hits the little cup three times, signaling another half hour of meditation. I look at the fishhook mark and try to open myself to enlightenment while also not thinking about it.

THE NEXT DAY, following a night spent on a cot in a tiled room shared with three other sesshin participants, I am awakened in the dark by someone ringing a bell outside my window. I stumble out the door to be shocked by the glittering closeness of the stars. It is four thirty in the morning. After breathing exercises on the patio beneath the zendo, we all troop upstairs for the first meditation session of the day. Several more sessions pass as I watch the mark in the wall in front of me turn from gray to yellow to white; then Fischer gives a dharma talk.

Dharma is translated from Sanskrit as "right behavior," and Fischer's dharma talks are roughly equivalent—in brevity and folksy tone if not in content—to the homily in a neighborhood Catholic church. In this one he says, "You could say that by studying Zen, we're studying the mind." But then he goes on, "There is a saying, 'A fingertip cannot touch itself. A knife cannot cut itself. A fire cannot burn itself.' And so a mind cannot understand itself. We cannot understand our consciousness because we *are* our consciousness. All we can do is live fully and joyfully in that consciousness." We can't understand it from the outside, either, Fischer says. "We can dissect the brain, and we can attach all kinds of machines to it, but these can only measure the *results* of consciousness; they cannot give a full understanding of it." And yet, of course, the goal of zazen is to understand consciousness, he says. To that end we are to try to open our minds to understanding. But "we cannot separate the body from the mind," he says. "You could not have a body without a mind or a mind without a body. So when we work on an open posture in zazen, it is to open our minds as well."

Weeks later, Fischer performs a reading of his poetry at Stanford. Afterward, no longer bound by the sesshin rule of silence, I ask him how exactly he thinks our posture might affect our brains. "Well," he says, "I'm not that focused on the brain myself." In his opinion, "to see the brain as somehow an independent agent is completely folly. I mean, what's the brain without the heart? What's the brain without the lungs? What's the brain without the circulatory system and the nervous system and the spinal column?" Of course, he says, "I'm not saying that the brain doesn't have a particular or important function within that system—it does. But I think that the toes are conscious. And that the fingertips make decisions and have knowledge. Not independently, but in association with the heart and the lungs and the liver and the brain." He goes on, "I mean, nobody's ever tried to transplant a brain. The body organs may be replaceable—all of them, possibly—and there would still be a sense of memory and identity."

Now, there is absolutely no scientific evidence to support the idea that your own brain isn't at least necessary (if not sufficient) for the particular mind that is yours. But Fischer is right: no one has ever done a brain transplant. If we ever learn how to keep a brain alive artificially and successfully attach it to another body's nervous system as we now hook transplanted hearts up to another body's circulatory system, we don't *know* what would happen. We are relying to some extent on the same kind of logic in our belief about the brain-mind connection that led Aristotle to assume a heart-mind connection: we just know that when the brain stops working, all evidence of the person it used to support goes away. At the moment, it is true, as Fischer says, that the brain is "part of a total system, and it can never be really and truly teased out of that system."

Many Western thinkers would agree with him on at least this part of his point. Even those who think it will be possible to make minds out of material other than neurons usually admit they won't be quite the same kind of minds as human minds, since all minds are dependent on the sensors bringing them information—in the case of humans, our skin, our eyes, our ears, our noses, the hormones floating throughout our bodies. It remains unclear how big a role our bodies play in our identity and how plastic that role is. But it seems impossible to imagine my particular mind unshaped by the sensation of cold water on my particular fingers, by my history of always being the shortest person in a room, by what I see when I look in the mirror. So as Fischer points out, despite the focus in Western science on our brains as the repositories and essence of our minds, those minds were created via the rest of our bodies, which can as easily be considered essential to our minds' existence.

Back in the zendo, Fischer wraps up the dharma talk with a description of Suzuki's teaching about breathing. According to Suzuki, your breath is like a swinging door between inside your body and outside it. There is unlimited space for your breath outside your body, he said, but also unlimited space for it inside the body. In this next round of zazen, we are to keep this idea in mind—while also, of course, letting go of it.

A COUPLE OF MONTHS after the sesshin, I drove north of San Francisco over the Golden Gate Bridge to Marin County to visit Fischer at the little one-bedroom apartment that serves as his office. The apartment is on the first floor of a two-story house at the top of a hill. I found Fischer there at his desk, writing documents in calligraphy for the ordination of a monk he would be performing the next day. When I arrived, he put away his brushes and ink and went into the tiny kitchen to make tea for us, which he knelt to serve me.

As we sipped it, Fischer told me about his life. "I always had, even as a child, a lot of questions about what is real and why do we have to die, et cetera," he said. As a boy, he began exploring some of those questions by writing poetry, a habit he continued as a philosophy major at Colgate University. While there, Fischer discovered Zen Buddhism, but he didn't practice or study it seriously. Later, at the Iowa Writers' Workshop, he found himself falling increasingly in love with language and its use but still unfulfilled—frustrated with his continued inability to answer or even successfully explore the big philosophic questions, and irritated with what he saw as the "re-hashed" nature of writing, the inevitability of writing about the past. It was then that he began to pursue Zen practice in earnest, searching for a new way to live and to write. Nevertheless it wasn't until he pursued a master's degree at the Graduate Theological Union in Berkeley that Fischer was finally able to meld his interests in Zen, philosophy, and language. He found that confluence in the teachings of Eihei Dogen, whose work served as the subject of his thesis. Dogen was not only a great writer, Fischer told me, but also wrote "in a particular way that was very much in keeping with the way that I was while I was studying Zen."

The way he was had something to do with a group of like-minded writers he had met around the time he arrived in Berkeley, who, he said, were "creating a very radical kind of avant-garde poetry that had to do with using language in very fractured and unusual ways." These were the language poets, a group that included Charles Bernstein, Lyn Hejinian, and Ron Silliman and that Fischer is occasionally classified as belonging to. Each was interested in the experience and creation of language itself—in exploring the full scope of what it is possible to say using language as well as testing language's limitations.

In short, seven hundred years after Dogen lived, Fischer and his friends were playing around with the same ideas he explored, and it is no wonder Fischer was drawn to him. When reading Dogen, "you know that he's talking about something very deep," Fischer said, "at the edge of what you can say in language." For instance, here is a passage from one of Dogen's philosophic works, known as *Uji*, which is translated as "The Time-Being":*

---

* This translation was done by Dan Welch and Kazuaki Tanahashi and appears in *Moon in a Dewdrop*, a collection and new translation of Dogen's work that Fischer also worked on.

Both mind and words are the time-being. Both arriving and not-arriving are the time-being. When the moment of arriving has not appeared, the moment of not-arriving is here. Mind is a donkey, words are a horse. Having-already-arrived is words and not-having-left is mind. Arriving is not "coming," not-arriving is not "not yet."

As Fischer found, philosophic questions about human experience inevitably bleed into questions about language and how it shapes, expresses, and limits that experience. There are many (including Daniel Dennett) who believe true human experience is impossible without language to mold and articulate it. Language is certainly universal among and specific to humans, although we still don't understand exactly why. Noam Chomsky argued more than thirty years ago that language must be innate, genetically hardwired into our brains, with all languages relying on a universal grammar with genetically encoded rules. In the decades since, linguists have been unable to find a set of syntactical rules that could be applied to all languages, and Chomsky himself appears to have softened on the idea of a heritable human grammar. Nevertheless the fact remains that humans, the creatures we are most sure are conscious, are also — as far as we can tell — the only ones with true language and the capacity for precise and subtle communication it affords. Even Sue Savage-Rumbaugh's bonobo Kanzi had a vocabulary of only two hundred symbols by the time he was six years old and was able to put together only rudimentary sentences to express himself. The average human child of six has a vocabulary of thirteen thousand words, meaning she has steadily learned one word every two to three hours since the age of two.

No one is even ready to guess at how much that voracious acquisition of language affects the development of our minds and experience. To what extent does language itself give us consciousness? And to what extent are we relying on language when we judge whether or not an entity is conscious? As Stickgold pointed out during his argument with Ned Block about the fusiform gyrus, how would we ever know if it were conscious in the absence of its ability to tell us about it?

And of course, even among those who can communicate with language, there is always the concern that what I say means something different to you than to me. The problem has particularly deep ramifications in the study of consciousness, as most of the data collected consist of reports of experience. David Chalmers, after describing his Hard Problem, actually raised the idea of creating another language (or refining our current one), allowing us to report experience more precisely. Would such a development simply push back the line between what we experience and what we are able to report? Or would it change our experience, expanding it to fit the new words used to describe it—or, in Orwellian fashion, limiting it by cutting out words open to interpretation? Would we even be able to learn, much less create, such a language?

During his Berkeley years, Fischer was trying to do what Chalmers would later suggest—to use language to precisely describe his experience and to study his own mind. The result was poems like this one, from a collection called *On Whether or Not to Believe in Your Mind:*

The Law

But are the steps not determined by the illness
The sensations, not the descriptions. And whatever you include
In thinking also in the middle of a train of thought
Say it was a picture (not a sensation, like hot) can't you
    Observe yourself and say "Who is doing this measuring?"
You expected this and that surprised you—what *kind*
Of a mistake was it? And is our confidence justified?
What would better relay it to us than success? Such as if you say
    "Fire has always burned me," are you
Just rounding things off? It *could* possibly remain in the air

And not fall, then he will see the light, it will

Dawn on him that "Aha! Now I have it!" but will he be able

    To go on after that?

Because, for instance, where else might he get to so suddenly?

A gesture of resignation.

All right then why not suppose thinking is always in a Language and

    The rules are sometimes in a Syntax

And the expression is tending toward a technique

Of a concept in a tradition.

Then you have to be too, slight, after all it won't do

    To make a false move. And what about memory & expressions

        like

A smile? Either you

Have this experience or you don't (to quote the law of the Excluded

    Middle

Fischer once wrote about Suzuki that "even when we do not precisely understand what he is getting at, we feel the truth and sincerity of what he is saying," and the same might be said about Fischer.

In addition to its capacity to shape and share our conscious experience, language enhances our minds' ability in another way. Sitting in his office, Fischer and I moved on to discuss a Zen story I had read. The Zen tradition is full of tales—not quite legends and not quite riddles—meant to provoke thought more than to provide concrete lessons for living, although they may do that as well. The one I had read describes a junior monk known to be a bookworm, who came across a passage that mentioned the possibility of a mustard seed's containing a mountain. The monk, named Li Bo, went to Zhishang, a wise senior monk, and asked how such a thing was possible. In response, Zhishang asked how ten thousand volumes could fit inside Li Bo's skull.

The story highlights another belief Fischer and Dennett share, which is that a good part of our minds are actually located not just outside our brains but outside our bodies. One of the great evolutionary triumphs that brought our minds to the level of sophistication we now enjoy was the ability to take up more and more information from our environment. But Dennett believes an even greater evolutionary leap came when we began to off-load information *to* our environment. He argues that, first through tools, which contain their instruction manuals within them by the nature of their design (he gives as an example, the self-explanatory hammer), and then through language, we have learned to manipulate the outside world in such a way that it serves as an extension of our minds.

For instance, on the index card where I wrote down the story of Li Bo and the mountain/mustard-seed paradox, I also wrote a symbol in the upper right-hand corner. That symbol directed me to another card listing the story's source (*Zen Speaks: Shouts of Nothingness*, a comic-book-style rendering of many Zen stories, written and illustrated by Tsai Chih Chung), which in turn leads to the book itself. The card, the symbol, and the book are all, in a sense, a part of my mind, Dennett would argue. They are also now part of yours. As he points out, in addition to allowing each of us access to information too vast to store in our own brains, humans' capacity to store information outside our bodies (in books, opera scores, photographs, MP3s, and so on) allows us to share that information with others, in effect blending our consciousnesses and allowing for parallel processing.

Fischer takes the idea one metaphysical step further, writing that "although our lives are located in our own hearts and minds, they are also located, perhaps most poignantly, in the space between us." Like Roberta Glick, he is an admirer of the Jewish theologian Martin Buber. "For Buber," he writes, "there is no God, no absolute, no present moment outside the profound relationship that takes place between the I and the you, between the self and the other. Within the hallowed reaches of that ineffable experience (which is not an experience, Buber insists) our true life takes place." In the same way, Fischer would argue, that a brain requires information and fuel from the body to support a mind, it also needs language and other people.

In his view, consciousness is bigger and more unified than Western thinkers give it credit for. Zen teaches that we are really all channeling the *same* consciousness, even though that's not how we experience it. "When we talk about 'my mind,'" he says, "we mean the conditioning, the condition lens, through which consciousness gets focused. And I call it my life." But really, he argues, we are all part of a universal consciousness, shared by all things. "DNA is consciousness, just the same as a cloud is consciousness, everything is consciousness," he says. "I recognize, of course, that there's a difference in degree between physical matter and sentient beings, but it's just this matter of degree, shades of difference, rather than any fundamental difference." And so, Fischer says, consciousness "has access at all points to all of reality—all that *is*," and thus "is not bound by conventional space-time notions." Time, he says, is a human construct and thus a part of human consciousness but not of the universal consciousness of which our consciousness is a part.

Both the idea that time is a human invention and the idea that consciousness is a matter of degree echo Dennett's thinking. In *Kinds of Minds* he argues that we are all guilty of what he calls "timescale chauvinism," a bias in favor of the speed at which we humans process and act. Invoking time-lapse photography to make his point, he writes, "See how that plant is striving upward, racing its neighbor for a favored place in the sun, defiantly thrusting its own leaves into the light, parrying the counterblows, ducking and weaving like a boxer!" He posits that part of the reason we don't usually credit trees with consciousness is simply that they are rooted in place and change so slowly.

Dennett uses the idea of timescale chauvinism to support his argument that the search for some clear division between conscious (or sentient) and not is futile. He himself tends not to talk seriously about consciousness having arisen until the evolution of brains, with their rapid associations and centralized control. But he writes that although "we do indeed have to draw lines across this multistranded continuum of cases, because having moral policies requires it," the idea that "we will *discover* a threshold—a morally significant 'step' in what is otherwise a ramp—is not only extremely unlikely but morally unappealing as well." Fischer agrees and thinks many of humanity's problems come from trying to find such steps in ramps.

ON THE MORNING of the last day of the sesshin, we are back in the zendo. It is December 8, the anniversary of the enlightenment of the Buddha. This is a *rohatsu* retreat to celebrate that day—*rohatsu* means "December eight" in Japanese. Outside, it seems there are butterflies everywhere, bright orange and yellow flutters against the green of the grass and palm fronds. The sky and water are different shades of the same intense blue, and the spume from the enormous crashing waves is like snow. At the morning dharma talk, Fischer tells us that this evening we will have a memorial service for the parents of a sesshin participant named Peter. Peter's parents died in the Holocaust: Both were taken to Auschwitz. His father was never heard from again; his mother survived and walked out of the camp, looking for Peter, a little boy at the time. She died before she could get to him.

The dharma talk is about genocide. Regarding the Holocaust, Fischer says, "It is so terrible it's almost impossible to believe it happened; it's almost as if the fabric of time were torn at that point in human history." He mentions the poet Paul Celan, who could only refer to the Holocaust, which he survived, as "that which happened." And so we come to what Fischer says are the problems he spends most of his time thinking about, the real reason he contemplates the mind. "Endemic human problems," he calls them, "like aggression, confusion, anger, alienation, inability to love—you know, all these human issues and problems. Fear of dying and so on. Fear of change, fear of life."

Fischer's life and way of thinking seem far removed from Glick's operating room, from Koch's lab, from Gabrieli's statistically analyzed brain scans, and certainly from playing Alpine Racer for Stickgold. But at heart the problems Fischer says he is working on constitute much of why we are fascinated by the human mind and consciousness. What we *really* want to know is why whoever shot Glick's patient did it. And if her patient somehow provoked it, why did he do the provoking? Work like Gabrieli's may someday explain what went wrong in Judy Castelli's brain, but will it ever lead to an understanding of how her abuser (or any child abuser, if you doubt her case) could do such horrible things to a child? When we wonder about our brains, aren't we wondering why they make us do what we do—why, despite the fact that they provide our capacity for logic, what we do is frequently illogical, counterproductive, or downright cruel? And why, despite our minds' awesome power to better our own lives, we are so frequently dissatisfied and unhappy to the point of being nasty to our loved ones, to the point of child abuse, war, and genocide?

Fischer thinks those are the real questions behind the drive to study the mind. And he believes meditation may both answer them and provide a solution to the problems raising them. He believes that through meditation we can somehow rise above or sink below or encompass more than human consciousness. By doing so, he believes we can escape both the bounds of time and the suffering we experience because of the way our particular human consciousness lenses bend the universal consciousness into such polarized notions as right and wrong, living and nonliving, conscious and not. Usually, he says, "we're focused on the lens as reality. We don't see that it's a lens through which we are perceiving it all; we think the lens is it. So we're stuck on a very narrow band of reality, thinking and identifying that as the totality of ourselves." Whereas, he says, "if I really understand and deeply enter a moment of my own experience, really and truly—I'm everywhere, I'm complete."

Despite the points where Fischer and Dennett seem to agree, I am sure Dennett would say that the lens *is* it, that consciousness arises within—absent any outside help or provenance—the complicated systems known as living things (and, potentially, complex man-made systems). Christof Koch, however, may be holding out for other possibilities as he struggles to reconcile his Catholicism with his life's work. When I met with him at Caltech, he told me he'd once given a talk on consciousness to a group of Catholic bishops. In that talk, he made the point that as far as science can tell, when your brain dies, your conscious mind dies. To his surprise, he told me, "They said, 'Yeah, we have no trouble with that.'" And in fact, one of the bishops made fun of the idea he said many of his parishioners held dear, that "the soul is like Casper the Ghost: when you die, it floats there up under the ceiling and Jesus plucks it out." According to Koch, the bishop said, "no, no, we know that's not the case. When you die, you're dead," but he went on, "However, at the end of time, God in his mercy resurrects you." Koch shrugged when he told me this, and said, "OK, now, science—there's nothing you can say about that, right? This is sort of beyond space-time causality."

I sometimes felt that of all my subjects, Judy Castelli would be the most likely to grasp Fischer's meaning when he describes our minds as lenses. Nevertheless, most of the others—Gabrieli and Glick, Crick and Stickgold and Illes—would agree that we simply don't know: it is at least possible that we are all just lenses for a vast, unified consciousness, with our brains' means of connecting to that consciousness still a mystery.

In one of his talks at the sesshin, Fischer said, "What you are doing here to your consciousness is like what people do to dough when they make bread. You are kneading it in order to make it soft and pliable." Fischer believes making our minds more pliable will allow us to practice compassion, make us able to deal with the pain (both physical and mental) in our lives without lashing out at other people — in short, that by meditating, we can make the world a better place.

That kind of belief is difficult for neuroscientists to swallow: What exactly does *pliable* mean? How can we think ourselves into health and happiness? Recently, however, there has been a surge of interest among Western scientists in how meditation affects the brain and the body. In 1992, Dr. Richard Davidson, based at the University of Wisconsin at Madison, began a series of functional-imaging studies on Tibetan Buddhist monks, who spend hours each day for years in meditation. Davidson, who calls himself an affective neuroscientist, had been studying the neuroscience of emotion for years. When he began studying the monks, he and other scientists had already shown, using EEG, that people in good moods or with generally happy temperaments tend to show more activity in their left prefrontal cortices than unhappy people.

Although he has yet to formally publish the results of his study of the monks' brains, Davidson has announced at conferences and in the popular press that one of the monks had the highest left prefrontal cortical activity of any subject he had ever scanned. That same monk was also apparently able to suppress his startle response. The startle response makes us jump (or at least blink) at the sound of a sudden loud noise and is accompanied by an increase in heart rate. When Davidson attempted to startle the monk with a loud noise, the monk reportedly didn't jump and didn't blink. Even his heart rate didn't respond to the stimulus. Such control was previously thought impossible.

There are a number of problems with such findings, which is likely why Davidson has yet to publish them: it's impossible to generalize from one subject, and even if all the monks he tested had increased activation in their left prefrontal cortices, we wouldn't know whether that extra activation was present before they started meditating. But Davidson has published another study that takes on some of those problems. He and his colleagues gathered forty-eight volunteers from a biotech company in Madison, Wisconsin. The researchers used EEG to measure the subjects' baseline brain activity, then randomized them into two groups. One group received two months of instruction and regular practice in a zazenlike mindfulness meditation technique, while the other group was put on a waiting list and given meditation training once the study was over. At the end of the eight weeks during which the experimental group meditated, the members of each group were again hooked up to the EEG. All subjects and controls were also given a flu vaccine at the end of the first group's meditation training period. Their blood was drawn one month and two months later and tested for antibodies to the vaccine.

Although the study was small and some of the measures failed to reach statistical significance, Davidson's experiment bore out Fischer's claims that meditation can improve our lives. The members of the group that had meditated now showed more left-side activation in their brains than the members of the control group. In questionnaires administered to both groups, the meditating group showed a decrease in anxiety over the eight weeks. The meditators also made significantly more antibodies in response to the flu shot than their nonmeditating counterparts. Other studies have shown that meditation can change levels of hormones in the blood and can lower blood pressure, reduce cholesterol levels and atherosclerosis, and lower the risk of death from cardiovascular disease. Western science cant't explain how, through meditation, we are able to change not only our minds but also our immune, endocrine, and cardiovascular systems. Such research, however, demonstrates that, as Fischer and other Buddhists have long believed, the mind-body connection is more complicated and tightly woven than Western thinkers have tended to allow, and that changes in the body and the mind may be more subject to our control than we realize.

In Fischer's view, the mystery of that relationship and of consciousness itself may never be solved, at least not by science. That he doesn't think science is the means by which we will understand it doesn't mean he thinks the scientific pursuit of such an understanding is a bad idea. Zen Buddhism, like empiric science, is based on the pursuit of truth and enlightenment, he said, and, as he has written, "We are human beings after all—wild and crazy beings!—earth tillers and star gazers—and we will never be satisfied without making the effort to know and live the truth."

| Sources

Introduction and Interludes

Braak, H., E. Braak, D. Yilmazer, and J. Bohl. 1996. Functional anatomy of human hippocampal formation and related structures. *J Child Neurol* 11(4): 265–75.

Burwell, R. D. 2000. The parahippocampal region: Corticocortical connectivity. *Ann N Y Acad Sci* 911: 25–42.

Dobelle, W. H. 2000. Artificial vision for the blind by connecting a television camera to the visual cortex. *Asaio J* 46(1): 3–9.

Feinberg, I. 1982. Schizophrenia: Caused by a fault in programmed synaptic elimination during adolescence? *J Psychiatr Res* 17(4): 319–34.

———. 1999. Mechanisms of hallucinations. *Am J Psychiatry* 156(5): 805–807.

Feinsod, M. 2001. Leeches for the unfortunate locksmith: Self-inflicted posttraumatic transient cerebral blindness—mode of treatment and underlying mechanism (1826). *Neurosurgery* 48(3): 660–63.

Gauthier, I., M. J. Tarr, A. W. Anderson, P. Skudlarski, and J. C. Gore. 1999. Activation of the middle fusiform "face area" increases with expertise in recognizing novel objects. *Nat Neurosci* 2(6): 568–73.

Geinisman, Y., L. de Toledo-Morrell, F. Morrell, I. S. Persina, and M. Rossi. 1992. Age-related loss of axospinous synapses formed by two afferent systems in the rat dentate gyrus as revealed by the unbiased stereological dissector technique. *Hippocampus* 2(4): 437–44.

Goetz, Christopher G. (ed.). 2003. *Textbook of Clinical Neurology*. 2nd ed. Philadelphia, Pa.: W. B. Saunders.

Green, J. B. 2003. Brain reorganization after stroke. *Top Stroke Rehabil* 10(3): 1–20.

Hoffman, R. E., and T. H. McGlashan. 1997. Synaptic elimination, neurodevelopment, and the mechanism of hallucinated "voices" in schizophrenia. *Am J Psychiatry* 154(12): 1683–89.

———. 1998. Reduced corticocortical connectivity can induce speech perception pathology and hallucinated "voices." *Schizophr Res* 30(2): 137–41.

———. 1999. Using a speech perception neural network simulation to explore normal neurodevelopment and hallucinated "voices" in schizophrenia. *Prog Brain Res* 121: 311–25.

———. 1999. Drs. Hoffman and McGlashan reply. *Am J Psychiatry* 156(5): 806–807.

———. 2001. Neural network models of schizophrenia. *Neuroscientist* 7(5): 441–54.

Holloway, M. 2003. The mutable brain. *Sci Am* 289(3): 78–85.

Huttenlocher, P. R. 1979. Synaptic density in human frontal cortex—developmental changes and effects of aging. *Brain Res* 163(2): 195–205.

Innocenti, G. M., F. Ansermet, and J. Parnas. 2003. Schizophrenia, neurodevelopment and corpus callosum. *Mol Psychiatry* 8(3): 261–74.

Kerkhoff, G. 2001. Spatial hemineglect in humans. *Prog Neurobiol* 63(1): 1–27.

Keshavan, M. S., S. Anderson, and J. W. Pettegrew. 1994. Is schizophrenia due to excessive synaptic pruning in the prefrontal cortex? The Feinberg hypothesis revisited. *J Psychiatr Res* 28(3): 239–65.

Levitt, Pat. 2003. Structural and functional maturation of the developing primate brain. *Journal of Pediatrics* 143 (4, Supplement 1): 35–45.

Margolis, R. L., D. M. Chuang, and R. M. Post. 1994. Programmed cell death: Implications for neuropsychiatric disorders. *Biol Psychiatry* 35(12): 946–56.

McGlashan, T. H., and R. E. Hoffman. 2000. Schizophrenia as a disorder of developmentally reduced synaptic connectivity. *Arch Gen Psychiatry* 57(7): 637–48.

Ott, P., and F. S. Larsen. 2004. Blood-brain barrier permeability to ammonia in liver failure: A critical reappraisal. *Neurochem Int* 44(4): 185–98.

Peters, A. 2002. Structural changes that occur during normal aging of primate cerebral hemispheres. *Neurosci Biobehav Rev* 26(7): 733–41.

Ragsdale, C. W., and E. A. Grove. 2001. Patterning the mammalian cerebral cortex. *Curr Opin Neurobiol* 11(1): 50–58.

Ramachandran, V. S., and Sandra Blakeslee. 1998. *Phantoms in the Brain*. New York: William Morrow and Co. Original edition, 1998.

Reddy, S., M. Zilvetti, J. Brockmann, A. McLaren, and P. Friend. 2004. Liver transplantation from non-heart-beating donors: Current status and future prospects. *Liver Transpl* 10(10): 1223–32.

Rhodes, G., G. Byatt, P. T. Michie, and A. Puce. 2004. Is the fusiform face area specialized for faces, individuation, or expert individuation? *J Cogn Neurosci* 16(2): 189–203.

Rossion, B., C. Schiltz, and M. Crommelinck. 2003. The functionally defined right occipital and fusiform "face areas" discriminate novel from visually familiar faces. *Neuroimage* 19(3): 877–83.

Sanes, Dan Harvey, Thomas A. Reh, and William A. Harris. 2000. *Development of the Nervous System*. San Diego, Calif.: Academic Press.

Selemon, L. D., G. Rajkowska, and P. S. Goldman-Rakic. 1995. Abnormally high neuronal density in the schizophrenic cortex. A morphometric analysis of prefrontal area 9 and occipital area 17. *Arch Gen Psychiatry* 52(10): 805–18; discussion 819–20.

Squire, Larry R. 2003. *Fundamental Neuroscience*. 2nd ed. Amsterdam; Boston: Academic Press.

Stanley, J. A., P. C. Williamson, D. J. Drost, T. J. Carr, R. J. Rylett, A. Malla, and R. T. Thompson. 1995. An in vivo study of the prefrontal cortex of schizophrenic patients at different stages of illness via phosphorus magnetic resonance spectroscopy. *Arch Gen Psychiatry* 52(5): 399–406.

Wijdicks, Eelco F. M. 2001. *Brain Death*. Philadelphia: Lippincott Williams and Wilkins.

Chapter 1: Touching the Brain

Conley, Frances K. 1998. *Walking Out on the Boys*. 1st ed. New York: Farrar, Straus and Giroux.

Croasdale, Myrle. 2004. Some Resident Work-Hour Limits Could Change: The ACGME Considers Raising 80–Hour Averages for a Few Specialties. American Medical Association, April 12, 2004 (cited May 11, 2004). Available from http://www.amaassn.org/amednews/2004/04/12/prse0412.htm.

Finger, Stanley. 1994. *Origins of Neuroscience: A History of Explorations into Brain Function*. New York: Oxford University Press.

Flitter, Marc. 1997. *Judith's Pavilion: The Haunting Memories of a Neurosurgeon*. 1st ed. South Royalton, Vt.: Steerforth Press.

Laws, E. R., Jr. 1999. Neurosurgery's man of the century: Harvey Cushing— the man and his legacy. *Neurosurgery* 45(5): 977–82.

Lewis, Sydney. 1994. *Hospital: An Oral History of Cook County Hospital*. New York: New Press. Distributed by W. W. Norton and Co.

Marx, John; Robert Hockberger (ed.); Ron Walls (ed.). 2002. *Rosen's Emergency Medicine: Concepts and Clinical Practice*. 5th ed. St. Louis: Mosby.

Penfield, Wilder. 1977. *No Man Alone: A Neurosurgeon's Life*. 1st ed. Boston: Little, Brown.

Sanderson, Mary Louise (Office Administrator, American Board of Neurosurgeons), personal communication, August 19, 2004.

Valenstein, Elliot S. 1986. *Great and Desperate Cures: The Rise and Decline of Psychosurgery and Other Radical Treatments for Mental Illness*. New York: Basic Books.

van Gijn, J. 2001. Camillo Golgi (1843–1926). *J Neurol* 248(6): 541–42.

Vertosick, Frank T. 1996. *When the Air Hits Your Brain: Tales of Neurosurgery*. New York: W. W. Norton.

Women in Neurosurgery. 2004. Women in Neurosurgery Web site 2000 (cited August 18, 2004). Available from http://www.neurosurgerywins.org/whoweare/certified.html.

Chapter 2: Watching the Brain

Brewer, J. B., Z. Zhao, J. E. Desmond, G. H. Glover, and J. D. Gabrieli. 1998. Making memories: Brain activity that predicts how well visual experience will be remembered. *Science* 281(5380): 1185–87.

Canli, T., J. E. Desmond, Z. Zhao, G. Glover, and J. D. Gabrieli. 1998. Hemispheric asymmetry for emotional stimuli detected with fMRI. *Neuroreport* 9(14): 3233–39.

Centers for Disease Control and Prevention. 2004. Symptoms of ADHD. CDC, February 4, 2004 (cited August 18, 2004). Available from http://www.cdc.gov/ncbddd/adhd/symptom.htm.

Cohen, L., S. Lehericy, C. Henry, M. Bourgeois, C. Larroque, C. Sainte-Rose, S. Dehaene, and L. Hertz-Pannier. 2004. Learning to read without a left occipital lobe: Right-hemispheric shift of visual word form area. *Ann Neurol* 56(6): 890–94.

Desmond, J. E., J. D. Gabrieli, A. D. Wagner, B. L. Ginier, and G. H. Glover. 1997. Lobular patterns of cerebellar activation in verbal working-memory and finger-tapping tasks as revealed by functional MRI. *J Neurosci* 17(24): 9675–85.

Desmond, J. E., J. M. Sum, A. D. Wagner, J. B. Demb, P. K. Shear, G. H. Glover, J. D. Gabrieli, and M. J. Morrell. 1995. Functional MRI measurement of language lateralization in Wada-tested patients. *Brain* 118 (pt. 6): 1411–19.

Dobbins, I. G., N. E. Kroll, E. Tulving, R. T. Knight, and M. S. Gazzaniga. 1998. Unilateral medial temporal lobe memory impairment: Type deficit, function deficit, or both? *Neuropsychologia* 36(2): 115–27.

Fernandez, G., J. B. Brewer, Z. Zhao, G. H. Glover, and J. D. Gabrieli. 1999. Level of sustained entorhinal activity at study correlates with subsequent cued-recall performance: A functional magnetic resonance imaging study with high acquisition rate. *Hippocampus* 9(1): 35–44.

Fernandez, G., A. Effern, T. Grunwald, N. Pezer, K. Lehnertz, M. Dumpelmann, D. Van Roost, and C. E. Elger. 1999. Real-time tracking of memory formation in the human rhinal cortex and hippocampus. *Science* 285(5433): 1582–85.

Fleischman, D. A., J. D. Gabrieli, D. W. Gilley, J. D. Hauser, K. L. Lange, L. M. Dwornik, D. A. Bennett, and R. S. Wilson. 1999. Word-stem completion priming in healthy aging and Alzheimer's disease: The effects of age, cognitive status, and encoding. *Neuropsychology* 13(1): 22–30.

Fleischman, D. A., J. D. Gabrieli, S. L. Reminger, C. J. Vaidya, and D. A. Bennett. 1998. Object decision priming in Alzheimer's disease. *J Int Neuropsychol Soc* 4(5): 435–46.

Fleischman, D. A., C. J. Vaidya, K. L. Lange, and J. D. Gabrieli. 1997. A dissociation between perceptual explicit and implicit memory processes. *Brain Cogn* 35(1): 42–57.

Gabrieli, J. D., J. B. Brewer, and R. A. Poldrack. 1998. Images of medial temporal lobe functions in human learning and memory. *Neurobiol Learn Mem* 70(1–2): 275–83.

Gabrieli, J. D., R. A. Poldrack, and J. E. Desmond. 1998. The role of left prefrontal cortex in language and memory. *Proc Natl Acad Sci U S A* 95(3): 906–13.

Gabrieli, J. D., C. J. Vaidya, M. Stone, W. S. Francis, S. L. Thompson-Schill, D. A. Fleischman, J. R. Tinklenberg, J. A. Yesavage, and R. S. Wilson. 1999. Convergent behavioral and neuropsychological evidence for a distinction between identification and production forms of repetition priming. *J Exp Psychol Gen* 128(4): 479–98.

Gould, Todd A. 2004. How MRI Works (Web site) (cited May 17, 2004). Available from http: //electronics.howstuffworks.com/mri.htm.

Park, S. M., J. D. Gabrieli, S. L. Reminger, L. A. Monti, D. A. Fleischman, R. S. Wilson, J. R. Tinklenberg, and J. A. Yesavage. 1998. Preserved priming across study-test picture transformations in patients with Alzheimer's disease. *Neuropsychology* 12(3): 340–52.

Poldrack, R. A., and J. D. Gabrieli. 1997. Functional anatomy of long-term memory. *J Clin Neurophysiol* 14(4): 294–310.

Poldrack, R. A., V. Prabhakaran, C. A. Seger, and J. D. Gabrieli. 1999. Striatal activation during acquisition of a cognitive skill. *Neuropsychology* 13(4): 564–74.

Prabhakaran, V., K. Narayanan, Z. Zhao, and J. D. Gabrieli. 2000. Integration of diverse information in working memory within the frontal lobe. *Nat Neurosci* 3(1): 85–90.

Ranganath, C., and K. A. Paller. 1999. Frontal brain activity during episodic and semantic retrieval: Insights from event-related potentials. *J Cogn Neurosci* 11(6): 598–609.

Rugg, M. D. 1998. Memories are made of this. *Science* 281(5380): 1151–52.

Rypma, B., V. Prabhakaran, J. E. Desmond, G. H. Glover, and J. D. Gabrieli 1999. Load-dependent roles of frontal brain regions in the maintenance of working memory. *Neuroimage* 9(2): 216–26.

Sobel, N., R. M. Khan, C. A. Hartley, E. V. Sullivan, and J. D. Gabrieli. 2000. Sniffing longer rather than stronger to maintain olfactory detection threshold. *Chem Senses* 25(1): 1–8.

Sobel, N., R. M. Khan, A. Saltman, E. V. Sullivan, and J. D. Gabrieli. 1999. The world smells different to each nostril. *Nature* 402(6757): 35.

Sobel, N., V. Prabhakaran, J. E. Desmond, G. H. Glover, R. L. Goode, E. V. Sullivan, and J. D. Gabrieli. 1998. Sniffing and smelling: Separate subsystems in the human olfactory cortex. *Nature* 392(6673): 282–86.

Sobel, N., V. Prabhakaran, C. A. Hartley, J. E. Desmond, Z. Zhao, G. H. Glover, J. D. Gabrieli, and E. V. Sullivan. 1998. Odorant-induced and sniff-induced activation in the cerebellum of the human. *J Neurosci* 18(21): 8990–9001.

Stebbins, G. T., J. D. Gabrieli, F. Masciari, L. Monti, and C. G. Goetz. 1999. Delayed recognition memory in Parkinson's disease: A role for working memory? *Neuropsychologia* 37(4): 503–10.

Straube, T., H. J. Mentzel, M. Glauer, and W. H. Miltner. 2004. Brain activation to phobia-related words in phobic subjects. *Neurosci Lett* 372(3): 204–208.

Thompson-Schill, S. L., J. D. Gabrieli, and D. A. Fleischman. 1999. Effects of structural similarity and name frequency on picture naming in Alzheimer's disease. *J Int Neuropsychol Soc* 5(7): 659–67.

Tulving, E. 1985. Memory and consciousness. *Can Psychol* 26(1): 1–12.

Tulving, E., and H. J. Markowitsch. 1998. Episodic and declarative memory: Role of the hippocampus. *Hippocampus* 8(3): 198–204.

Tversky, B., and E. J. Marsh. 2000. Biased retellings of events yield biased memories. *Cognit Psychol* 40(1): 1–38.

Unattributed. 2004. Time Traveller Goes Back to 1987 (Web site), July 19, 1998 (cited February 24, 2004). Available from http://www.100megsfree4.com/farshores/p_time.htm.

Wagner, A. D., J. E. Desmond, G. H. Glover, and J. D. Gabrieli. 1998. Prefrontal cortex and recognition memory. Functional-MRI evidence for context-dependent retrieval processes. *Brain* 121(pt. 10): 1985–2002.

Wagner, A. D., G. T. Stebbins, F. Masciari, D. A. Fleischman, and J. D. Gabrieli. 1998. Neuropsychological dissociation between recognition familiarity and perceptual priming in visual long-term memory. *Cortex* 34(4): 493–511.

Zacks, J., B. Rypma, J. D. Gabrieli, B. Tversky, and G. H. Glover. 1999. Imagined transformations of bodies: An fMRI investigation. *Neuropsychologia* 37(9): 1029–40.

Chapter 3: Mining the Brain

Antal, A., E. T. Varga, M. A. Nitsche, Z. Chadaide, W. Paulus, G. Kovacs, and Z. Vidnyanszky. 2004. Direct current stimulation over MT+/V5 modulates motion aftereffect in humans. *Neuroreport* 15(16): 2491–94.

Crick, Francis. 1994. *The Astonishing Hypothesis: The Scientific Search for the Soul.* New York: Simon and Schuster (Touchstone).

———. 1996. Visual perception: Rivalry and consciousness. *Nature* 379(6565): 485–86.

Crick, F., and C. Koch. 1998. Consciousness and neuroscience. *Cereb Cortex* 8(2): 97–107.

———. 2003. A framework for consciousness. *Nat Neurosci* 6(2): 119–26.

DeAngelis, G. C., and W. T. Newsome. 1999. Organization of disparity-selective neurons in macaque area MT. *J Neurosci* 19(4): 1398–415.

Engstrom, A. 2003. Presentation Speech—Nobel Prize in Physiology or Medicine. Elsevier Publishing Company 1962 (cited October 28, 2003). Available from http://www.nobel.se/medicine/laureates/1962/press.html.

Fried, I., C. L. Wilson, K. A. MacDonald, and E. J. Behnke. 1998. Electric current stimulates laughter. *Nature* 391(6668): 650.

Kamitani, Y., and F. Tong. 2005. Decoding the visual and subjective contents of the human brain. *Nat Neurosci* 8(5): 679–85.

Koch, Christof. 2003. *The Quest for Consciousness.* Denver, Colo.: Roberts and Company.

Kohn, A., and J. A. Movshon. 2003. Neuronal adaptation to visual motion in area MT of the macaque. *Neuron* 39(4): 681–91.

Kornberg, Arthur. 2003. The Biologic Synthesis of Deoxyribonucleic Acid (Web site). Elsevier Publishing 1959 (cited October 28, 2003). Available from http: //www.nobel.oo/medicine/laureates/1959/kornberg lecture .pdf.

Kreiman, G., I. Fried, and C. Koch. 2002. Single-neuron correlates of subjective vision in the human medial temporal lobe. *Proc Natl Acad Sci USA* 99(12): 8378–83.

Kreiman, G., C. Koch, and I. Fried. 2000. Imagery neurons in the human brain. *Nature* 408(6810): 357–61.

———. 2000. Category-specific visual responses of single neurons in the human medial temporal lobe. *Nat Neurosci* 3(9): 946–53.

Maugh, Thomas H. 2002. Vision of the future: Researchers are on the right track to produce artificial sight for the blind. *Los Angeles Times*, September 16.

Nichols, M. J., and W. T. Newsome. 2002. Middle temporal visual area microstimulation influences veridical judgments of motion direction. *J Neurosci* 22(21): 9530–40.

Orgel, Leslie E. 2004. Molecular Biology: Retrospective: Francis Crick (1916–2004). *Science* 305(5687): 1118.

Rose, D. 1996. Some reflections on (or by?) grandmother cells. *Perception* 25(8): 881–86.

Sacks, Oliver. 2004. In the River of Consciousness. *New York Review of Books*, January 15.

Sagon, Candy. 2003. Cakey vs. fudgy. *Washington Post*, October 8, F01.

Salzman, C. D., C. M. Murasugi, K. H. Britten, and W. T. Newsome. 1992. Microstimulation in visual area MT: Effects on direction discrimination performance. *J Neurosci* 12(6): 2331–55.

Sanders, Robert. 2003. Nobelist James Watson headlines Berkeley symposium on DNA and biotech (Web site). UCBerkeley News, October 13, 2003 (cited October 13, 2003). Available from http: //www.berkeley.edu/ news/media/releases/2003/10/13_dna.shtml.

Unattributed. 2003. Francis Crick—Biography (Web site). Elsevier

Publishing Co., June 27, 2003 (cited October 29, 2003). Available from http: //www.nobel.se/medicine/laureates/1962/crick-bio.html.

———. 2003. At night, why does it take my eyes several minutes to get used to darkness? (Web site). HSW Media Network (cited December 8, 2003). Available from http: //www.howstuffworks.com/question53.htm.

———. 2003. A Visit with Dr. Francis Crick (Web site). Access Excellence @ the National Health Museum 1989 (cited October 28, 2003). Available from http: //www.accessexcellence.org/AE/AEC/CC/crick.html.

———. 2003. Brain myths (editorial). *Nat Neurosci* 6(2): 99.

Watson, J. D., and F. H. Crick. 2003. Molecular structure of nucleic acids: A structure for deoxyribose nucleic acid. *Am J Psychiatry* 160(4): 623–4.

Wellman, H. M., D. Cross, and J. Watson. 2001. Meta-analysis of theory-of-mind development: The truth about false belief. *Child Dev* 72(3): 655–84.

Chapter 4: The Dreaming Brain

Bertolo, H., T. Paiva, L. Pessoa, T. Mestre, R. Marques, and R. Santos. 2003. Visual dream content, graphical representation and EEG alpha activity in congenitally blind subjects. *Brain Res Cogn Brain Res* 15(3): 277–84.

Campbell, S. S., and I. Tobler. 1984. Animal sleep: A review of sleep duration across phylogeny. *Neurosci Biobehav Rev* 8(3): 269–300.

Jan, J. E., and P. K. Wong. 1988. Behaviour of the alpha rhythm in electroencephalograms of visually impaired children. *Dev Med Child Neurol* 30(4): 444–50.

Kemerling, Garth. 2004. Aristotle: Logical Methods (Web site), October 27, 2001 (cited February 18, 2004). Available from http: //www.philosophy pages.com/hy/2n.htm.

Nolte, John. 1999. *The Human Brain: An Introduction to Its Functional Anatomy*. 4th ed. St. Louis: Mosby.

Office of Communications and Public Liaison, and National Institute of Neurological Disorders and Stroke. 2004. Understanding Sleep: Brain Basics (Web site). NINDS/NIH, July 3, 2003 (cited June 3, 2004). Available from http: //www.ninds.nih.gov/health_and_medical/pubs/

understanding_sleep_brain_basic_.htm#Sleep: %20A%20Dynamic%20 Activity.

Stickgold, R., J. A. Hobson, R. Fosse, and M. Fosse. 2001. Sleep, learning, and dreams: Off-line memory reprocessing. *Science* 294(5544): 1052–57.

Stickgold, R., A. Malia, D. Maguire, D. Roddenberry, and M. O'Connor. 2000. Replaying the game: Hypnagogic images in normals and amnesics. *Science* 290(5490): 350–53.

Stickgold, R., D. Whidbee, B. Schirmer, V. Patel, and J. A. Hobson. 2000. Visual discrimination task improvement: A multi-step process occurring during sleep. *J Cogn Neurosci* 12(2): 246–54.

Tranel, D., and A. R. Damasio. 1988. Non-conscious face recognition in patients with face agnosia. *Behav Brain Res* 30(3): 235–49.

Unattributed. 2004. Game-Revolution (Web site) (cited January 20, 2004). Available from http://www.game-revolution.com/download/pc/action/ carmageddon.htm.

Walker, M. P., T. Brakefield, A. Morgan, J. A. Hobson, and R. Stickgold. 2002. Practice with sleep makes perfect: Sleep-dependent motor skill learning. *Neuron* 35(1): 205–11.

Walker, M. P., T. Brakefield, J. Seidman, A. Morgan, J. A. Hobson, and R. Stickgold. 2003. Sleep and the time course of motor skill learning. *Learn Mem* 10(4): 275–84.

Chapter 5: Multiple Minds

American Psychiatric Association. 2000. *Diagnostic and Statistical Manual of Mental Disorders—Fourth Edition (Text Revision)*. 4th ed. Washington, D.C.: American Psychiatric Association.

Anderson, M. C., K. N. Ochsner, B. Kuhl, J. Cooper, E. Robertson, S. W. Gabrieli, G. H. Glover, and J. D. Gabrieli. 2004. Neural systems underlying the suppression of unwanted memories. *Science* 303(5655): 232–35.

Janet, Pierre. 2004. *An Autobiography of Pierre Janet* (Web site). Republished by Christopher D. Green, York University, with permission of Clark University Press, Worcester, Mass. (original publishers), March 2000

(1930) (cited February 5, 2004). Available from http://psychclassics
.yorku.ca/Janet/murchison.htm.

Kahn, R. J., and P. G. Kahn. 1997. The medical repository—the first U.S.
medical journal (1797–1824). *N Engl J Med* 337(26): 1926–30.

Kenny, M. G. 1998. Disease process or social phenomenon? Reflections on
the future of multiple personality. *J Nerv Ment Dis* 186(8): 449–54.

Kosslyn, S. M., W. L. Thompson, M. F. Costantini-Ferrando, N. M. Alpert,
and D. Spiegel. 2000. Hypnotic visual illusion alters color processing in
the brain. *Am J Psychiatry* 157(8): 1279–84.

Lewis, D. O., C. A. Yeager, Y. Swica, J. H. Pincus, and M. Lewis. 1997. Objective documentation of child abuse and dissociation in 12 murderers
with dissociative identity disorder. *Am J Psychiatry* 154(12): 1703–10.

Merskey, H. 1995. Multiple personality disorder and false memory syndrome. *Br J Psychiatry* 166(3): 281–83.

Mitchill, S. L. 1816. A double consciousness, or a duality of person in the
sane individual. *The Medical Repository* 3: 185–86.

Nakatani, Y. 2000. Dissociative disorders: From Janet to DSM-IV. *Seishin
Shinkeigaku Zasshi* 102(1): 1–12.

Ross, C. A. 1995. Multiple personality disorder and false memory syndrome.
Br J Psychiatry 167(2): 263–64; author reply 265–66.

Sar, V., L. I. Yargic, and H. Tutkun. 1996. Structured interview data on 35
cases of dissociative identity disorder in Turkey. *Am J Psychiatry* 153(10):
1329–33.

Spanos, N. P., J. R. Weekes, E. Menary, and L. D. Bertrand. 1986. Hypnotic
interview and age regression procedures in the elicitation of multiple
personality symptoms: A simulation study. *Psychiatry* 49(4): 298–311.

Spiegel, D., and E. Cardena. 1991. Disintegrated experience: The dissociative disorders revisited. *J Abnorm Psychol* 100(3): 366–78.

Thigpen, Corbett H., and Hervey M. Cleckley. 1957. *The Three Faces of Eve.*
New York: McGraw-Hill.

Tsai, G. E., D. Condie, M. T. Wu, and I. W. Chang. 1999. Functional magnetic resonance imaging of personality switches in a woman with dissociative identity disorder. *Harv Rev Psychiatry* 7(2): 119–22.

Chapter 6: Mind and Magic

Ariyasu, H., K. Takaya, T. Tagami, Y. Ogawa, K. Hosoda, T. Akamizu, M. Suda, T. Koh, K. Natsui, S. Toyooka, G. Shirakami, T. Usui, A. Shimatsu, K. Doi, H. Hosoda, M. Kojima, K. Kangawa, and K. Nakao. 2001. Stomach is a major source of circulating ghrelin, and feeding state determines plasma ghrelin-like immunoreactivity levels in humans. *J Clin Endocrinol Metab* 86(10): 4753–58.

Bliss, T. V., and G. L. Collingridge. 1993. A synaptic model of memory: Long-term potentiation in the hippocampus. *Nature* 361(6407): 31–39.

Block, Ned. 1997. Anti-reductionism slaps back. *Mind, Causation, World, Philosophical Perspectives* 11: 107–133.

Brook, Andrew, and Don Ross. 2002. *Daniel Dennett, Contemporary Philosophy in Focus*. Cambridge; New York: Cambridge University Press.

Dennett, Daniel. 1991. *Consciousness Explained*. 1st ed. Boston: Little, Brown and Co.

———. 1993. Review of *The Rediscovery of Mind* by John Searle. *Journal of Philosophy* 60(4): 193–205.

———. 1996. *Kinds of Minds: Toward an Understanding of Consciousness*. 1st ed. New York: Basic Books.

———. 1998. *Brainchildren: Essays on Designing Minds, Representation and Mind*. Cambridge: MIT Press.

———. 2003. Autobiographical essay. *Philosophy Now* (forthcoming).

Hofstadter, Douglas R., and Daniel Clement Dennett. 1981. *The Mind's I: Fantasies and Reflections on Self and Soul*. New York: Basic Books.

Malenka, R. C. 2003. The long-term potential of LTP. *Nat Rev Neurosci* 4(11): 923–26.

Nagel, Thomas. 1974. What is it like to be a bat? *Philosophical Review* LXXXIII (October 4): 435–50.

Orr, H. Allen. 2004. A Passion for Evolution. Review of *A Devil's Chaplain: Reflections on Hope, Lies, Science, and Love*. *New York Review of Books*, February 26.

Searle, John R. 1999. Consciousness (Web site). Available from http://ist-socrates.berkeley.edu/~jsearle/articles.html (accessed May 16, 2004).

Shermer, Michael. 2004. None so blind. *Sci Am* (March) 42.

Simons, D. J., and C. F. Chabris. 1999. Gorillas in our midst: Sustained inattentional blindness for dynamic events. *Perception* 28(9): 1059–74.

Williams, Robert Hardin et al. 2002. *Williams Textbook of Endocrinology.* 10th ed. Philadelphia, Pa.: W. B. Saunders.

Chapter 7: Open Mind

BrightHouse Institute for Thought Sciences. 2004. BrightHouse Institute for Thought Sciences Launches First "Neuromarketing" Research Company Company Uses Neuroimaging to Unlock the Consumer Mind (Web site). PRWeb 2002 (cited February 9, 2004). Available from http: //www.prweb.com/releases/2002/6/prweb40936.php.

———. 2004. Clients, Achievements and Recognition. BrightHouse 2003 (cited February 21, 2004). Available from http: //www.thoughtsciences. com/clients.html.

Burton, H. 2003. Visual cortex activity in early and late blind people. *J Neurosci* 23(10): 4005–11.

Butcher, J. 2003. Cognitive enhancement raises ethical concerns. Academics urge pre-emptive debate on neurotechnologies. *Lancet* 362(9378): 132–33.

Canli, T., Z. Zhao, J. E. Desmond, E. Kang, J. Gross, and J. D. Gabrieli. 2001. An fMRI study of personality influences on brain reactivity to emotional stimuli. *Behav Neurosci* 115(1): 33–42.

Editors, *Scientific American.* 2003. SA perspectives: A vote for neuroethics. *Scientific American* 289(3): 13.

Ganis, G., S. M. Kosslyn, S. Stose, W. L. Thompson, and D. A. Yurgelun-Todd. 2003. Neural correlates of different types of deception: An fMRI investigation. *Cereb Cortex* 13(8): 830–36.

Illes, J. 2003. Neuroethics in a new era of neuroimaging. *American Journal of Neuroradiology* 24(9): 1739–41.

Illes, J., and M. Kirschen. 2003. New prospects and ethical challenges for neuroimaging within and outside the health care system. *American Journal of Neuroradiology* 24(10): 1932–34.

Illes, J., J. E. Desmond, L. F. Huang, T. A. Raffin, and S. W. Atlas. 2002.

Ethical and practical considerations in managing incidental findings in functional magnetic resonance imaging. *Brain Cogn* 50(3): 358–65.

Illes, J., E. Fan, B. A. Koenig, T. A. Raffin, D. Kann, and S. W. Atlas. 2003. Self-referred whole-body CT imaging: Current implications for health care consumers. *Radiology* 228(2): 346–51.

Illes, J., M. P. Kirschen, and J. D. Gabrieli. 2003. From neuroimaging to neuroethics. *Nat Neurosci* 6(3): 205.

Illes, J., and T. A. Raffin. 2002. Neuroethics: An emerging new discipline in the study of brain and cognition. *Brain Cogn* 50(3): 341–44.

Johansson, B. B. 2004. Brain plasticity in health and disease. *Keio J Med* 53(4): 231–46.

Jones, H., J. Illes, and W. Northway. 1995. A history of the Department of Radiology at Stanford University. *AJR Am J Roentgenol* 164(3): 753–60.

Kaiser, C. P. 2004. Feds Fail to Stop fMRI Marketing Studies (Web site). DiagnosticImaging.com, CMP Media LLC, February 17, 2004 (cited February 21, 2004). Available from http://www.diagnosticimaging.com/dinews/2004021701.shtml.

Kim, B. S., J. Illes, R. T. Kaplan, A. Reiss, and S. W. Atlas. 2002. Incidental findings on pediatric MR images of the brain. *AJNR Am J Neuroradiol* 23(10): 1674–77.

McClure, S. M., J. Li, D. Tomlin, K. S. Cypert, L. M. Montague, and P. R. Montague. 2004. Neural correlates of behavioral preference for culturally familiar drinks. *Neuron* 44(2): 379–87.

Mokhiber, Russell, and R. Weissman. 2004. Bayer Makes Worst Corporations List for 2003 (February 13, 2004) (Web site). *Berkeley Daily Planet*, February 13, 2004 (cited February 22 2004). Available from http://www.berkeleydaily.org/article.cfm?archiveDate=02–13–04&storyID=18266.

———. 2004. Multiple Corporate Personality Disorder: The 101 Worst Corporations of 2003 (vol. 24, no. 12) (Web site). Multinational Monitor 2004 (cited February 22, 2004). Available from http://multinationalmonitor.org/mm2003/03december/dec03corp1.html.

Moseley, M., R. Bammer, and J. Illes. 2002. Diffusion-tensor imaging of cognitive performance. *Brain Cogn* 50(3): 396–413.

Pasquale, S. A., T. J. Russer, R. Foldesy, and R. S. Mezrich. 1997. Lack of interaction between magnetic resonance imaging and the copper-T380A IUD. *Contraception* 55(3): 169–73.

Potenza, M. N., M. A. Steinberg, P. Skudlarski, R. K. Fulbright, C. M. Lacadie, M. K. Wilber, B. J. Rounsaville, J. C. Gore, and B. E. Wexler. 2003. Gambling urges in pathological gambling: A functional magnetic resonance imaging study. *Arch Gen Psychiatry* 60(8): 828–36.

Rojo, A., M. Aguilar, M. T. Garolera, E. Cubo, I. Navas, and S. Quintana. 2003. Depression in Parkinson's disease: Clinical correlates and outcome. *Parkinsonism Relat Disord* 10(1): 23–28.

Rushkoff, Douglas. 2004. Reading the Consumer Mind: The Age of Neuromarketing Has Dawned (Volume 17, Issue 7) (Web site). New York Press 2004 (cited February 21, 2004). Available from http: //www.nypress.com/17/7/news%26columns/rotation.cfm.

Sample, I., and D. Adam. 2003. The brain can't lie. *The Guardian*, November 20, 4.

Taylor, A. J., and P. G. O'Malley. 1998. Self-referral of patients for electron-beam computed tomography to screen for coronary artery disease. *N Engl J Med* 339(27): 2018–20.

Thompson, Clive. 2003. There's a sucker born in every medial prefrontal cortex. *New York Times*, October 26, 54.

Unattributed. 2004. Body Scan Scams, Black Boxes in Cars, and More (Web site). Tech TV 2003 (cited February 8, 2004). Available from http: //www.techtv.com/news/shownotes/story/0,24195,3526772,00.html.

———. 2004. Commercial Alert Asks Feds to Investigate Neuromarketing Research at Emory University (Web site) 2003 (cited February 21, 2004). Available from http: //www.commercialalert.org/index.php/category_id/1/subcategory_id/82/article_id/211.

———. 2004. Emerging field of neuromarketing. In *Weekend All Things Considered*. USA: NPR.

———. 2003. A vote for neuroethics. *Scientific American* 289(3): 13.

Wahlberg, David. 2004. Advertisers probe brains, raise fears (Web site). *Atlanta Journal-Constitution* (cited February 21, 2004). Available from http: //www.commercialalert.org/index.php/external/true/article_id/214.

Chapter 8: Mind and Body

Austin, James H. 1998. *Zen and the Brain: Toward an Understanding of Meditation and Consciousness.* Cambridge: MIT Press.

Cai, Zhizhong, and Brian Bruya. 1994. *Zen Speaks: Shouts of Nothingness.* New York: Anchor Books.

Chalmers, David. 2004. How Can We Construct a Science of Consciousness? In *The Cognitive Neurosciences, III,* edited by M. Gazzaniga. Cambridge: MIT Press.

Davidson, R. J., J. Kabat-Zinn, J. Schumacher, M. Rosenkranz, D. Muller, S. F. Santorelli, F. Urbanowski, A. Harrington, K. Bonus, and J. F. Sheridan. 2003. Alterations in brain and immune function produced by mindfulness meditation. *Psychosomatic Medicine* 65(4): 564–70.

Dennett, Daniel. 1994. The Role of Language in Intelligence. In *What Is Intelligence,* edited by J. Khalfa. Cambridge: Cambridge, Cambridge Univ. Press.

Downing, Michael. 2001. *Shoes Outside the Door: Desire, Devotion, and Excess at San Francisco Zen Center.* Washington, D.C.: Counterpoint.

Dumoulin, Heinrich. 1963. *A History of Zen Buddhism.* New York: Pantheon Books.

Fields, Rick. 1992. *How the Swans Came to the Lake: A Narrative History of Buddhism in America.* 3rd ed. Boston, Mass.: Shambhala Publications.

Front, Robert. 2004. Interview with Norman Fischer. *Jack Magazine* 1996 (cited June 25, 2004). Available from http://www.jackmagazine.com/issue2/path.html.

Gethin, Rupert. 1998. *The Foundations of Buddhism.* Oxford: Oxford University Press.

Goleman, Daniel. 2003. *Destructive Emotions: How Can We Overcome Them?: A Scientific Dialogue with the Dalai Lama.* New York: Bantam Books.

Gyatso, Tenzin (His Holiness the 14th Dalai Lama), H. C. Cutler, 1998. *The Art of Happiness.* New York: Riverhead Books.

Hall, Stephen S. 2003. Is Buddhism good for your health? *New York Times,* September 14, 46.

Hyman, Carol. 2005. A Meeting of the Minds: Buddhists and Behavioral Scientists Compare Notes on the Workings of the Mind (Web site).

UC Berkeley Media Relations 2003 (cited March 7, 2005). Available from http://ihd.berkeley.edu/keltnernews11-4-03.htm.

Johnson, George. 1995. Chimp talk debate: Is it really language? *New York Times*, June 6, 1995, 1.

Kaminski, J., J. Call, and J. Fischer. 2004. Word learning in a domestic dog: Evidence for "fast mapping." *Science* 304(5677): 1682-3.

Katagiri, Dainin, and Steve Hagen. 1998. *You Have to Say Something: Manifesting Zen Insight*. 1st ed. Boston: Shambhala.

Kim, D. H., Y. S. Moon, H. S. Kim, J. S. Jung, H. M. Park, H. W. Suh, Y. H. Kim, and D. K. Song. 2005. Effect of Zen meditation on serum nitric oxide activity and lipid peroxidation. *Prog Neuropsychopharmacol Biol Psychiatry* 29(2): 327-31.

Olson, Carl. 2000. *Zen and the Art of Postmodern Philosophy: Two Paths of Liberation from the Representational Mode of Thinking*. Albany: State University of New York Press.

Searle, John R. 2002. End of the revolution. Review of *New Horizons in the Study of Language and Mind*. *New York Review of Books*, February 28.

Storlie, Erik Fraser. 1996. *Nothing on My Mind: Berkeley, LSD, Two Zen Masters, and a Life on the Dharma Trail*. 1st ed. Boston: Shambhala.

Suzuki, Daisetz Teitaro, and Zenchu Sato. 1965. *The Training of the Zen Buddhist Monk*. New York: University Books.

Suzuki, Shunryu, and Trudy Dixon. 1970. *Zen Mind, Beginner's Mind*. 1st ed. New York: Walker/Weatherhill.

Tooley, G. A., S. M. Armstrong, T. R. Norman, and A. Sali. 2000. Acute increases in night-time plasma melatonin levels following a period of meditation. *Biol Psychol* 53(1): 69-78.

Unattributed. 1987. *The Holy Teaching of Vimalakirti: A Mahayana Scripture*. Translated by R.A.F. Thurman: Pennsylvania State University Press.

———. 2005. Joy Detectives (Web site). Windhorse Publications (cited March 7, 2005). Available from http://www.dharmalife.com/issue21/joydetectives.html.

Walton, K. G., R. H. Schneider, and S. Nidich. 2004. Review of controlled research on the transcendental meditation program and cardiovascular disease. Risk factors, morbidity, and mortality. *Cardiol Rev* 12(5): 262-66.

| Illustration Credits

Unless otherwise noted, all illustrations are reprinted from Henry Gray, *Anatomy of the Human Body*, 20th ed., revised and edited by Warren H. Lewis (Philadelphia: Lea and Febiger, 1918).

Page 4: Reprinted from T. Sadler, *Langman's Embyrology*, 9th ed. (Philadelphia: Lippincott Williams and Wilkins, 2003), pp. 93 and 95, with permission from Lippincott Williams and Wilkins.

Page 11: Drawing by Ramon y Cajal reprinted with permission from Ramon y Cajal's heirs.

Page 39: Reprinted from Sanes et al., *Development of the Nervous System*, 1st ed. (Philadelphia: Elsevier, 2000), p. 85, with permission from Elsevier.

Pages 63 and 74: Reprinted from Sanes et al., *Development of the Nervous System*, 1st ed. (Philadelphia: Elsevier, 2000), p. 155, with permission from Elsevier.

Page 94: Reprinted from Christof Koch, *The Quest for Consciousness* (Greenwood Village, CO: Roberts and Company, 2004), p. 270, with permission from Roberts and Company and the author.

Page 100: Rendered by Shannon Moffett; adapted with permission from Vince Di Lollo.

Page 110: Reprinted from Kandel et al., *Principles of Neural Science,* 3rd ed. (Appleton and Lange, 1996), p. 23, with permission from McGraw-Hill Companies.

Page 166: Reprinted from S. M. Kosslyn, W. L. Thompson, M. F. Costantini-Ferrando, N. M. Alpert, and D. Spiegel, "Hypnotic Visual Illusion Alters Color Processing in the Brain," *American Journal of Psychiatry* 157:1279–1284, August 2000, with permission from the authors.

Page 181: Drawing by Judy Castelli reprinted from the personal collection of the artist with permission.

Page 188: Reprinted from Kandel et al., *Principles of Neural Science,* 3rd ed. (Appleton and Lange, 1996), p. 19, with permission from McGraw-Hill Companies.

| Index

abuse of children, 171–72, 174, 175–76, 178, 273

Accreditation Council for Graduate Medical Education, 30n

action potentials, 187–89

adolescence, brain development during, 144–46

adulthood, changes in the brain in, 184–89

"After Apple–Picking," 123

aging, brain function and, 222–26
  declarative memory, 222, 224–26
  executive function, 222–24

agnosics, 133–34

allergies, 119

alpha waves, 126–27

Alpine Racer, 111–12, 121, 132

Alzheimer's disease, 225–26, 236

American Academy of Neurology, 254

American Psychiatric Association, 152

amnesia and amnesiacs, 59–60, 61, 62
  sleep experiments with, 124, 125, 126

a.m/p.m. experiments, 92

amygdala, 55, 89

anatomy of the brain, 4–6, 20–21

aneurysms, 21

antibiotics, 16, 17

antidepressants, 236

arachnoid, 20

archicortex, 6

Aristotle, 68–69, 118, 264

ascending reticular activating system, 120

Associated Professional Sleep Societies, 137

Association for the Scientific Study of Consciousness, 75–76, 191

Astonishing Hypothesis, The (Crick), 69

astrocytes, 109, 110

attention, 211–13

attention deficit/hyperactivity
  disorder, 236
auditory priming, 61
automatic acts, 152–53
axons, 11, 63–64, 74, 109–10, 188, 189

Baars, Dr. Bernard, 76
bacitracin, 36
backward masking, 101
Basbaum, Dr. Allan, 2–3
behaviorism, 76
Bell Laboratories, 52
Benadryl, 119
Berkeley Daily Planet, 244
Bernstein, Charles, 266
beta-amyloid protein, 225
Bianchi, Kenneth (Hillside
  Strangler), 162–63
binocular rivalry, 95
blindness, 15, 99
  brain reorganization and, 177, 249
blindsight, 81
Block, Dr. Ned, 212–14, 216, 268
blood-brain barrier, 17–18, 109, 119
body scanning, self-referred, 231–32,
  233–34, 252
BOLD (blood-oxygen-level
  dependent) technique, 52
bone wax, 36
bonobos, study of communication by,
  84–86, 251, 267
brain, see specific subjects related to the
  brain
brain abscess, 17, 18–19, 21
brain stem, 255
  functions of, 6, 18

brain tumors, 9–10, 21
breathing, 265
BrightHouse, 241–44, 251
Buber, Martin, 270

California Institute of Technology
  (Caltech), Koch's lab at, 86–87,
  90–92, 96
cancer, 52
  brain tumors, 9–10
  of pituitary gland, 15
Caplan, Arthur, 240–41
"Cartesian Theater," 194, 196, 210
Castelli, Judy, 147–49, 150, 153–58,
  161–62, 165, 169–71, 174, 178,
  179–83, 227, 273, 274
Cavendish Laboratory, 72–73
Celan, Paul, 272
cerebellum, function of, 6
cerebral cortex, 6, 39, 109
cerebral hemispheres, 5–6
cerebrospinal fluid (CSF), 20, 21, 39
Chalmers, Dr. David, 190, 218, 221,
  268
change blindness, 149
Chase, Truddi, 159
child abuse, 171–72, 174, 175–76, 178,
  273
childhood, brain development
  during, 109–10
Chomsky, Noam, 86, 267
Churchland, Paul, 217
"cinematographic vision" after brain
  damage, 103
circadian clock, 120
Cleckley, 159

cognitive neuroscience, 45, 46, 52–53
  meanings of words, changing,
    135–37
Cohen, Dr. Neal, 59
Commercial Alert, 244
Conley, Dr. Frances, 31
consciousness, 66
  attention and, 211–13
  Crick and Koch's framework for
    studying, 78–84, 99, 101, 104–105
  Crick and Koch's research on, 69,
    73–84, 86–105
  Dennett's Fame in the Brain,
    model for, 203–205, 208–209, 211
  evolution and, 214–15
  the Hard Problem, 190, 191, 221
  increase in research on, 76–77
  ineffable aspects of, 218–19
  information storage outside our
    bodies, 270
  "layered" nature of, 99
  line between not-conscious and,
    213–16
  more than one, *see* dissociative
    identity disorder (DID)
  neural correlates of (NCC), *see*
    neural correlates of
    consciousness (NCC)
  of other living creatures, 84–85
  sense of seamlessness of, 102–104
  universal, 271
  Zen Buddhism and, 257–77
Consciousness Explained (Dennett),
    194, 196–97, 206, 209–10
consumer behavior, fMRI research
  on, 241–45

Cooper, Dr. Leon, 202
Corkin, Dr. Suzanne, 53
"cortical reflexes" ("zombie modes"),
    81, 82, 88
craniotomy, 19, 22–23, 88
Crick, Francis, 66–83, 99–108, 113,
    190, 196, 202, 229n, 248
Crick, Odile, 66, 68, 102, 105–108
criminal justice system, functional
    neuroimaging and, 247–50
Cushing, Dr. Harvey, 22

Damasio, Antonio, 133, 134, 228, 248
Dana Foundation, 227
Darwin's Dangerous Idea (Dennett),
    194
Davidson, Dr. Richard, 275–76
daydreams, 137
death, defining the concept of,
    253–56, 274
declarative forms of memory, 60, 125,
    140–41
  aging and, 222, 224–26
  changes over time, 141
  sleep and, 142
delta waves, 129
dendrites, 11, 63, 64, 75, 188
  spines, 74
Dennett, Dr. Daniel, 68, 190–221,
    248, 249, 260, 267, 269–70,
    271–72, 274
Dennett, Susan, 199
depression, 236
Descartes, René, 194–96, 198
Descartes' Error (Damasio), 228
developmental biology, 73

development of the brain
  in adolescence, 144–46
  in adulthood, 184–89
  in childhood, 109–10
  death, 253–56
  embryonic period, 39–42
  in fetal period, 63–65
  in old age, 222–26
  postconception, 4–6
dharma, 263
*Diagnostic and Statistical Manual of
  Mental Disorders* (American
  Psychiatric Association), 152, 159,
  161
diapedesis, 17
diffusion, 17, 186
Dilbert, Terry, case of, 44, 45, 56, 140,
  141
Di Lollo, Dr. Vince, 100
dissociation, 152
  trauma and, 153
dissociative identity disorder (DID),
  147–83
  cases reported in medical literature,
    150–52, 159, 175–76
  Castelli case, *see* Castelli, Judy
  confused with schizophrenia, 154, 169
  defined, 152
  Dennett on, 209–10
  hypnotically induced, 162–64, 167
  as legal defense, 161
  skeptics questioning existence of,
    160–61, 162, 167, 178–79, 182–83
  trauma and stress and, 160, 171–73
DNA, discovery of structure of, 66,
  72–73, 108, 113–14, 229n

Dogen, Eihei, 257, 266–67
dopamine, 145
Double Helix, The (Watson), 67
dreaming and sleep, *see* sleep and
  dreaming
dualism, 196–97, 260
dura matter, 20–21, 24

Edelman, Dr. Gerald, 202
EEG (electroencephalography), 77,
  126–27, 254, 275, 276
Ehrlich, Paul, 17
Einstein, Albert, 42
electroculogram, 126
electromyogram, 126
embolus, 24–25
embryonic period, brain development
  in, 39–42
Emory University, 242, 244–45
emotions, electrical stimulation of the
  brain and change in, 98–99
entorhinal cortex, 225
epileptic seizures, neurosurgery to
  alleviate, 54–55, 89, 124n
ethics, 228
  of neuroscience, 227–52
evolution, 207, 208, 214–15
executive functioning, 173, 174, 250
  aging and, 222–24
eyewitness testimony, false memories
  and, 247

face recognition, 40, 42, 46, 63,
  132–33, 134
"Facing Up to the Problem of the
  Consciousness," 190

Feeling of What Happens, The
  (Damasio), 133n, 228
Feinberg, Dr. Irwin, 145, 146
fetal period of brain development,
  63–65
50 First Dates, 56n
Fischer, Norman, 111, 257–77
flash suppression, 94, 96
foramen magnum, 17
forgetting, 172–77
fornix, 56
forward masking, 101
"Framework for Consciousness, A,"
  78–83, 99, 101, 104–105
Franklin, Rosalind, 73
Freud, Sigmund, 62, 153
  repression, 174
Fried, Dr. Itzhak, 89–94, 96, 98, 99
From a Logical Point of View (Quine),
  198
frontal lobe, 5, 15
Frost, Robert, 123
functional magnetic resonance
  imaging (fMRI), 47, 53, 61, 62,
  67, 76, 83, 121, 236–40
  Alzheimer's disease, to diagnose,
    226, 236
  depression and antidepressants,
    research on, 236
  dissociative identity disorder
    (DID) study, 159–60
  future uses in popular culture,
    240–45
  limits of, 77–78
  neuroethics and, 233–35, 240–45
  principles behind, 47–49, 52

psychiatric evaluation, use in, 252
raw data from, interpreting,
  239–40
self-referred, 233, 234–35
fusiform gyrus, 40, 42, 63, 132–33, 171,
  213, 268

Gabrieli, Dr. John, 2, 43–62, 66,
  172–73, 211, 228, 233, 273
Gage, Phineas T., 223, 243, 248
galvanic skin response, 133, 134
Geller, Uri, 217
General Electric, 48
genetic determinism, 248–49
Gerasimov, Vadim, 122
glial cells, 109–10
Glick, Dr. Roberta, 7–38, 176, 257
Glover, Dr. Gary, 48–49, 52, 53,
  236–37
Goldman, Edwin, 17
Golgi, Camillo, 12, 200n
grandmother cells, 90, 92, 96
*Greater Magic: A Practical Treatise on
  Modern Magic* (Hilliard), 220
Greely, Henry, 249, 250–51
Guthrie, Woody, 114

hallucinations, schizophrenia and, 145
Hard Problem, 190, 191, 221
Hebb, Donald, 200
Hejinian, Lyn, 266
hemispherectomies, 38
hemorrhagic stroke, 24, 25, 37–38
heterophenomenology, 218
"higher levels first," concept of,
  99–100

Hill, Anita, 31, 32
Hilliard, John, 220–21
hippocampus, 89, 133, 160, 173, 225, 247
    epileptic seizures and, 54–55, 124n
    memory consolidation and, 55–56,
      141
histamine, 119, 120
HM (patient used in memory
    studies), 54–62, 141
Hobson, Allan, 116
Hofstadter, Douglas, 207
hormone production, sleep and,
    117–18
Hull, Ralph W., 192–93, 220
Huntington's disease, 114
Huttenlocher, Dr. Peter, 144, 145
hypnosis, 152, 153, 162–67, 183
    defining, 164–65
hypothalamus, 14
    histamine release and sleep, 119, 120
    vegetative state and, 255

Illes, Judy, 228–36, 239–41, 245, 251, 252
imagining, areas of the brain
    activated by, 94
immune system, 189n
    sleep and, 117
intelligence, brain size and, 42
ischemic stroke, 24–25

James, William, 47–48
Janet, Pierre, 152–53, 171
Jewish mysticism, 10
Jung, Carl, 153
justice system, functional
    neuroimaging and, 247–50

Kanzi (bonobo), 84–85, 86, 251, 267
K complexes, 128, 129
Kerrison rongeurs, 23
Kierkegaard, Soren, 233
Kinds of Minds (Dennett), 271
Kirschen, Matt, 77, 233, 237–39, 240
Koch, Christof, 43, 66–108, 126, 190,
    191–92, 196, 216, 219–20, 251,
    274
Kolers, Paul, 206n
Kreiman, Gabriel, 91

language, 267–68, 270, 271
lateral prefrontal cortex, 173
learning
    during adolescence, 146
    associative networks of neurons
      and, 200
    dendrite spines and, 74
    sleep and, 138–40, 142
learning disorders, 46
Lettvin, Dr. Jerome, 90
Lewis, Dr. Dorothy Otnow, 175–76
lie-detector tests, 133
limbic lobe, 5
liquefactive necrosis, 18

magic, 216–21
magnetic resonance imaging (MRI),
    47, 48, 237
    fetuses and newborns, scanning of,
      235
    spin and, 49–50
    theory behind, 49–51
    see also functional magnetic
      resonance imaging (fMRI)

*Man Who Mistook His Wife for a Hat,
The* (Sacks), 103
marketing, fMRI research used for,
241–45, 251
meaning, 105
Meaux, Dr. Justine, 242, 355
Medical Research Council, England,
72
medical residents, sleep deprivation
of, 140n
meditation, 258, 259, 263, 273, 275, 276
Meditations (Descartes), 198
MEG (magnetoencephalography),
77
memory, 53, 135, 209
consolidation of memories, 44–45,
55–56, 139, 140–43
declarative forms of, *see* declarative
forms of memory
false memories, 178, 246–48
HM (patient used in memory
studies), 54–62
loss of, Dilbert case and, 44, 45,
56
misattribution, 246–47
multiple memory systems theory,
45, 58–60
nondeclarative forms of, *see*
nondeclarative forms of memory
Schacter's seven sins of, 245–46
"source," 224
suppression, 172–77
tricking, by association, 246–47
mental illness, fMRIs for diagnosis
of, 236
Milner, Dr. Brenda, 53–54, 58–59

mind
conscious, *see* consciousness
unconscious, *see* unconscious
mind-enhancing drugs, 230
mirror drawing, 59, 125
Mitchill, Samuel Latham, 150–52, 159
molecular biology, 71, 73, 248
monkeys
aging and prefrontal cortex, 224
study of visual systems of, 84, 96–97
Montague, Dr. P. Read, 242–45
morphogens, 40
Mosso (Italian physician), 47–48
motion, perception of, 102–104
motion aftereffect, 102
motor cortex, 40, 41
motor skills, learning of, 139–40
Multinational Monitor, 244
multiple personality disorder, *see*
dissociative identity disorder
(DID)
multiple sclerosis, 189n
myelin, 110, 144, 188–89, 224

Nader, Ralph, 244
Nagel, Dr. Thomas, 218
Nature, 73
Nature Neuroscience, 78, 79
Necker cube, 94–95
neocortex, 6, 142
Net of Magic (Siegel), 216
neural correlates of consciousness
(NCC), 75–76, 104–105, 191
Koch's experiments, 89–95
neural plasticity, 249–50
neural progenitor cells, 39, 108

neural tube, 4–5, 39, 40
neurodeterminism, 249
neuroeconomics, 245
neuroessentialism, 251
neuroethics, 227–52
"Neuroethics: Mapping the Field,"
    227–28, 229, 230, 240, 241,
    245–46, 249
neurofibrillary tangles, 225
neuromarketing, 241–45, 251
Neuron, 242
neurons, 39, 199–201
    axons, 11, 63–64, 74, 109–10, 188, 189
    cell body, 64
    cell membrane, 184–88
    "coalitions" of, 82, 104, 199–201, 211
    dendrites, *see* dendrites
    "guideposts," 64
    Hebb's hypothesis, 200–201
    Koch's experiments on visual
        perception and individual, 89–95
    "organizers," 40
    penumbras of the, 105
    storage of information and, 82
    synapses, *see* synapses
    synchronized firing of, 104–105
    transplanting of human, into mice,
        250–51
    see also development of the brain
neurosurgeons
    female, gender discrimination and,
        30, 31–33
    training required of, 30
neurosurgery, 7–8, 16, 19–24
    for epileptic seizures, 54–55, 89
    for gunshot wound to the head,
        16–17, 19–24, 33–34, 35–37

hemispherectomies, 38
historically, 22
postoperative survival, 35
recovery from, 14
Neurosurgery, 32
neurotransmitters, 189
    receptors for, 65
    release of, 65
    reuptake of, 109, 189
"New Crossroads: Neuroimaging and
    Neuroethics," 233
Newsome, Dr. William, 2, 96–97
Nightcap, 124, 125
nondeclarative forms of memory, 59,
    60–62, 125
    priming and, 60–62
    sleep and learning skills requiring,
        139–40, 142

occipital cortex, 165
occipital lobe, 5, 15
Office for Human Research
    Protections, 244–45
Olby, Robert, 72
olfaction, 46, 62
oligodendrocytes, 109–10, 188, 189n
*On Whether or Not to Believe in Your
    Mind* (Fischer), 268
optic chiasm, 14, 15, 120
optic nerves, 14, 15
optic tract, 14, 15

pain
    dura matter and, 20
    as subjective, 2
paleocortex, 6
Panbanisha (bonobo), 85–86, 251

parahippocampal gyrus, 247
Paranormal Pages, 44
parietal lobe, 5
Parkinson's disease, 236
Pavlovski, Dmitri, 122
Pazhitnov, Alexey, 122
Penfield, Wilder, 41
phi, 205–206
philosophical writings on
    consciousness, 76
    see also individual authors and titles
Physics (Aristotle), 118
pia matter, 20
pineal gland, 194–95
pituitary gland, 14, 15, 119
planning, 214, 224
    see also executive functioning
plasticity of the brain, 176–77
Poggio, Dr. Tomaso, 73–74, 75
polygraph tests, 133
polysomnographs, 121, 126–27, 128
positron-emission tomography
    (PET), 52, 165, 248
postconception development of the
    brain, 4–6
post-traumatic stress disorder, 160
Potter, Van Rensselaer, 229
prefrontal cortex, 222–24, 241n, 243
    lateral, 173
    left, 275
"Preserved Learning and Retention
    of Pattern-Analyzing Skill in
    Amnesia: Dissociation of
    Knowing How and Knowing
    That," 59
primates, nonhuman, consciousness
    of, 84–86

priming, 60–62
Prince, Morton, 159
Principia Mathematica (Russell and
    Whitehead), 114, 118
Principles of Psychology (James),
    47–48
prison inmates with dissociative
    identity disorder (DID), study
    of, 175–76
privacy issues, 245, 247
prosopagnosia, 134

qualia, 79–80, 134
Quest for Consciousness, The (Koch), 83
Quian-Quiroga, Dr. Rodrigo, 90n
Quine, Willard, 198, 199

radial glia, 39, 109
Radiology, 230–31
Ramachandran, V. S., 176
Ramón y Cajal, Dr. Santiago, 200
Randi, James "the Amazing," 217
Reddy, Leila, 90n
REM sleep, 130–32, 137, 139
Reynolds, Mary, 150–52, 159
Robert Wood Johnson Medical
    School, 237
Ryle, Gilbert, 199

Sacks, Dr. Oliver, 103
Safire, William, 227–28, 229
sagittal section, 54
Salk Institute, 73
San Francisco Chronicle, 31
Savage-Rumbaugh, Dr. Sue, 84–86,
    267
Schacter, Dr. Daniel, 245–47

schizophrenia, 145, 154, 169, 236
Schreiber, Flora Rheta, 159
Science, 59, 125
Scientific American, 114, 230
Scoville, Dr. William, 54, 55, 89
Searle, Dr. John, 76, 219
self, concept of, Dennett's view of, 210
self-referred body scanning, 231–32,
    233–34, 252
semaphorins, 64
sensing, 214
Siddhartha Gautama, 261–62
Siegel, Lee, 216–17
Silliman, Ron, 266
Simons, Dr. Daniel, 149–50, 211, 212
simultaneous masking, 101
skull, 6, 17, 21
sleep and dreaming, 111–43
   during adolescence, 146
   attempts to discover reasons for,
     117–19, 138–40, 142–43
   defining dreaming, 137–38
   histamine and, 119, 120
   hormone production and, 117–18
   immune system and, 117
   learning and, 138–40
   movement during, 130–31
   stages of, 128–32, 146
sleep spindles, 129, 138–39
Smith, Dr. Vernon, 245
somatotopic map of the brain, 41
Sominex, 119
Song, Dr. Mike, 7, 13, 15, 19–24,
    33–34, 35, 36–37, 140n
Soto Buddhists, 259
Spanos, Dr. Nicholas, 162–64, 167

Spiegel, Dr. David, 159, 160, 165–69,
    178, 181, 182
spinal cord, 18, 20
   postconception development of, 4
spirituality, science and, 32–33
Squire, Dr. Larry, 59, 60
standardized brain, 238
Stanford University, 53, 96
   Center for Biomedical Ethics,
    229
   Gabrieli's lab at, 45–47, 236
startle response, 275
stem-cell research, 250
Stickgold, Dr. Bob, 112–43, 147, 171,
    178–79, 213, 251, 267–68
   sleep lab, 112–13
stress and dissociative identity
    disorder (DID), 160
stroke
   hemorrhagic, 24, 25, 37–38
   ischemic, 24–25
subconscious, 152–53
superior sagittal sinus, 21, 36, 37
suprachiasmatic nucleus of the
    hypothalamus, 120
surgery, brain, *see* neurosurgery
Suzuki, Shunryu, 260–61, 265, 269
Switzer, Dr. Paul, 93
Sybil, 158–59, 161
synapses, 63, 64, 65, 109
   age and synaptic pruning process,
    144–45, 146, 224
synaptic cleft, 65, 189

tau (protein), 225
Tech TV, 233, 236

temporal lobe, 5, 54
  medial, 89, 160
Tetris, 121–22, 123–26, 137
thalamus, 6, 14–15, 121
  sensory information and, 121
theory of mind, 85
Thigpen, 159
Thomas, Clarence, 31, 32
Thomson, Dr. Donald, 246
Tibetan Buddhism, 275
time, as human construct, 271
trauma
  dissociation and, 153
  dissociative identity disorder
    (DID) and, 160, 171–73
trephinations, 22
tuberomamillar nucleus of the
  hypothalamus, 119, 120
Tulving, Endel, 60
"Tuned Deck, The" (magic trick),
  192–93, 219–22
Turn Left in Order to Go Right
  (Fischer), 259

Uji (Dogen), 266–67
unconscious(ness), 81
  sleep and, 117, 118
  Freud and, 62
uncus, 55
University of California at Los
  Angeles, School of Medicine, 89

vegetative state, 255–56
Vertosick, Dr. Frank, 13

video games as research tools, 111–12,
  121–26, 132, 137
visual agnosias, 133
visual masking, 100–101
visual systems, 15, 75, 81–84
  of monkeys, study of, 84, 96–97
  "movie in your brain," 102–104
  multiple, 81–82
  research on, 81–84, 89–102
von Grunau, Michael, 206n
voxels, 77, 239

Walking Out on the Boys (Conley),
  32
Washington Post, 68
waterfall effect, 102
Watson, Dr. James, 66, 67, 72–73, 108,
  113, 229n
Weinberg, Steven, 108
Weissman, Dr. Irving, 250–51
Wertheimer, Max, 206n
"What Is It Like to Be a Bat?", 218
What Mad Pursuit (Crick), 71
Wilbur, Cornelia, 159
Wilkins, Maurice, 73
Wittgenstein, Ludwig, 134
Women in Neurosurgery, 31

Zen Buddhism, 257–77
Zen Mind, Beginner's Mind (Suzuki),
  260
zombie modes, see "cortical reflexes"
  ("zombie modes")